Spirituality in Mind

Spirituality in Mind

Psychiatry in a Post-Secular Age

Christopher C. H. Cook
Durham University

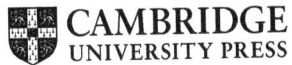
CAMBRIDGE
UNIVERSITY PRESS

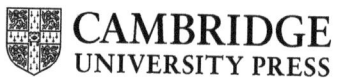

Shaftesbury Road, Cambridge CB2 8EA, United Kingdom

One Liberty Plaza, 20th Floor, New York, NY 10006, USA

477 Williamstown Road, Port Melbourne, VIC 3207, Australia

314–321, 3rd Floor, Plot 3, Splendor Forum, Jasola District Centre, New Delhi – 110025, India

Cambridge University Press is part of Cambridge University Press & Assessment, a department of the University of Cambridge.

We share the University's mission to contribute to society through the pursuit of education, learning and research at the highest international levels of excellence.

www.cambridge.org
Information on this title: www.cambridge.org/9781009629171

DOI: 10.1017/9781009629201

First published 2026

Cover image: Guang Cao /Moment / Getty Images

A catalogue record for this publication is available from the British Library

A Cataloging-in-Publication data record for this book is available from the Library of Congress

ISBN 978-1-009-62917-1 Paperback

Cambridge University Press & Assessment has no responsibility for the persistence or accuracy of URLs for external or third-party internet websites referred to in this publication and does not guarantee that any content on such websites is, or will remain, accurate or appropriate.

For EU product safety concerns, contact us at Calle de José Abascal, 56, 1°, 28003 Madrid, Spain, or email eugpsr@cambridge.org

....

Every effort has been made in preparing this book to provide accurate and up-to-date information that is in accord with accepted standards and practice at the time of publication. Although case histories are drawn from actual cases, every effort has been made to disguise the identities of the individuals involved. Nevertheless, the authors, editors, and publishers can make no warranties that the information contained herein is totally free from error, not least because clinical standards are constantly changing through research and regulation. The authors, editors, and publishers therefore disclaim all liability for direct or consequential damages resulting from the use of material contained in this book. Readers are strongly advised to pay careful attention to information provided by the manufacturer of any drugs or equipment that they plan to use.

This book is dedicated to my grandparents, only one of whom I knew as an adult, and two of whom died before I was born:
Christopher and Alice Cook, and William and Ethel Holland.

The good leave an inheritance to their children's children.

(Proverbs 13:22)

Contents

Acknowledgements

Having edited two editions of *Spirituality and Psychiatry* and having enjoyed enormously working with authors who brought to each of these volumes a wide range of experience, knowledge and perspectives on the subject, I realise that there are nonetheless some things that cannot be achieved in an edited multi-author volume. In light of this experience, the present book offers a personal perspective on the field, drawing on academic and clinical work in different contexts over several decades. It could not have been written but for numberless conversations I have had with colleagues and patients over the years, both in person and in print, and for the many mentors, teachers and others who shaped my formation as a psychiatrist, priest and academic. It is an impossible task to list them all here and I fear that, in mentioning some, I shall later regret not mentioning others. However, my fellow editors of *Spirituality and Psychiatry*, Andrew Sims and Andrew Powell, and the other contributors to those books certainly rank highly in the list of those to whom I am in debt.

Spirituality and Psychiatry was originally conceived as a project of the Spirituality and Psychiatry Special Interest Group (SPSIG) at the Royal College of Psychiatrists (RCPsych). My thinking about many of the issues in the present book has been shaped by fellow members of the executive committee, and by delegates and speakers at our many day conferences (and, more recently, webinars). I am especially grateful to Andrew Sims who, in his term as chair, invited me to join the SPSIG executive well over 20 years ago.

I owe much to a one-time fellow medical student at St George's Hospital Medical School, now a professor of psychiatry, Rob Poole, who takes a different view to me on the place of spirituality in psychiatry and has always held me to account for what I write and say on the topic (and who will quite likely disagree with much of what I have written in this book!). Thank you, Rob, for disagreeing with humour and goodwill and for helping me to see things differently. You haven't converted me, but you have helped me to think more critically.

I have had the privilege of working for a number of NHS trusts in different parts of the country, and the case studies in this book draw on almost all of them. I am particularly indebted to colleagues and patients with whom I have worked in the spirituality engagement group of the Tees, Esk and Wear Valleys NHS Foundation Trust, of which I am still a member. This group, which includes patients, chaplains and multidisciplinary medical colleagues, has provided a safe space within which we have been able to think together, and to think creatively, about how best to address the spiritual needs of patients and staff in clinical practice and service delivery.

I have learnt so much about the medical humanities from colleagues at Durham University, not least the important concept of entanglement, which I have taken up in this book. A big thank-you therefore goes to Angela Woods, current director of the Institute for Medical Humanities in Durham, and to all my past and present colleagues in IMH.

I would like to express special gratitude to Jessica Papworth at Cambridge University Press, who consistently encouraged me to submit a proposal for this book, steered me through the commissioning process and patiently talked through the many permutations of titles that were proposed. Along with the rest of the team at the Press, she has been a consistent source of helpful advice and publishing wisdom.

Thank you to the anonymous (and some not so anonymous) peer reviewers who offered constructive feedback on the original proposal and accompanying draft chapters, and on the submitted final draft of the manuscript of this book. Thank you to Gwen Adshead and Toby Howarth, who read parts of the book in draft form and offered feedback. Thank you to Hanneke Schaap-Jonker, who kindly sent me copies of several of her papers and one of her books, when I was in correspondence with her about the research literature on God image for Chapter 4. Thanks also to Bruno Mosqueiro for his advice on the Brazilian Psychiatric Association guidelines discussed in Chapter 8.

Most of the case studies are composites and none are published here under the real names of those involved. However, I'm enormously grateful to 'Jenny' and 'Sarah', and to the many patients and others whose personal stories have, directly or indirectly, contributed to this book. There is a popular misunderstanding that people learn to be doctors at medical school, whereas in fact we learn, and go on learning, most of what really matters vocationally and professionally from our patients (and similar things might be said about clergy) long after we have supposedly 'qualified'.

Introduction

Psychiatry in a Post-Secular Age

This is a book about psychiatry. A lot of books about psychiatry, even by psychiatrists, tend to foreground its difficulties, controversies and detractions. Thomas Szasz (1962) notoriously, and with apparently little understanding of the positive role of myth in human well-being, questioned the very existence of psychiatry in *The Myth of Mental Illness.*[1] Anthony Clare's book was famously about *Psychiatry in Dissent* (Clare, 1980). More recently, Tom Burns (2014) has written about *Our Necessary Shadow* and Ben Cave (2023) about *What We Fear Most.* My friend Gwen Adshead, a forensic psychiatrist, referring to her work with patients who are also offenders, wrote about *The Devil You Know* (Adshead and Horne, 2021). In conversation with some critics of psychiatry, it can feel as though it is psychiatrists themselves who are the devils, and yet psychiatry is dedicated to helping others, and to bringing healing and recovery from the suffering of mental illness.

Following in this tradition of psychiatrists writing about psychiatry, I am also seeking to draw attention to one of the issues over which psychiatry is 'in dissent', and, although – unlike Szasz – I think that the concept of mental illness is a useful one in pursuit of relieving human distress, I am also wanting to question some of the fundamental assumptions that psychiatry makes. We have lots of dissent, not least in relation to the place of spirituality in psychiatry, and yet we too often do not look as critically as we might at the assumptions that we make, as psychiatrists, about psychiatry and about what it is that our patients really want from us. Like our patients, we have our shadows and our fears. We are human beings too, and this influences the ways in which we go about our work. I see this not as a fatal flaw but, rather, as an all too often unrealised asset.

This book proposes a positive vision of the core concerns of psychiatry as understood through the lens of spirituality. It is not about what we fear most – it is about what we desire most. Although I will talk about the metaphorical shadows, because it is the task of psychiatry to address them, my aim is to say more about the light that casts them. Of course, our fears and our desires, shadows and light, are not unrelated. We fear that we will lose, or fail to find, what we desire. The opposite of what we value most highly may be experienced as a 'necessary shadow' or may be demonised. A focus on signs and symptoms of illness is a natural tendency of medicine, since our patients come to us asking for help with their problems, which we traditionally refer to as their 'presenting complaints'. However, most of them are not complaining, they are seeking recovery. They do not want their lives to be focussed on what has gone wrong; they want to be well. Psychiatry, I am suggesting, should have this positive goal of human flourishing firmly in mind when making

---

[1] This was followed by later books including, with an even more unsubtle title, *Psychiatry: The Science of Lies* (Szasz, 2008).

a diagnosis or developing a treatment plan. This positive therapeutic endeavour is, I suggest, inextricably connected with spirituality.

Spirituality and Psychiatry

This book is about spirituality and psychiatry. There have been a large number of such books over recent years, and it may well be asked why we need another one. My first answer to that question is that many of the other, very excellent, books (e.g., Huguelet and Koenig, 2009; Moreira-Almeida et al., 2021) focus primarily on the science. Whilst I will address the scientific research evidence here, and the empirical evidence base is important, I believe that we need to be much more interdisciplinary in engagement with perspectives from the humanities, especially theology and religious studies. Scientific research on spirituality and psychiatry has often focussed on what is most easily measurable rather than what is most meaningful; I'm hoping to redirect our attention to the spiritual quest for meaning.

Secondly, my intention is to show that spirituality is not an optional extra, or something that has simply been neglected, or even something that has statistical significance and so should be taken more seriously; rather, it actually *is* a core concern of psychiatry. When psychiatry appears to be ignoring spirituality, or excluding it, or when voices are heard pleading that it should not be forgotten, what has actually happened is that psychiatry has adopted a particular theological stance – an 'atheology'. Psychiatry is not, and never has been, neutral or disinterested in relation to spirituality and religion. Rather, it has imposed a pragmatic atheism which is so much taken for granted that it has become virtually invisible, except to those patients for whom it causes distress. My aim in this book is to make these invisible assumptions visible in order that they may be critically reconsidered.

Spirituality and religion are notoriously difficult terms to define, and we shall consider their contested utility in Chapter 1. They are important, insofar as this book is concerned, because they refer, however imprecisely, to aspects of human experience and meaning-making which are perceived as deeply important to most people worldwide. Even in more secular Western countries, amongst which the UK ranks highly, there are many who consider themselves spiritual but not religious (SBNR) (Mercadante, 2014) and yet others who might not identify as spiritual or religious but for whom key aspects of spirituality (e.g., transcendent relationships, meaning and purpose in life) are still very important. Many others continue to find traditional religious ways of belonging and believing vital to expressing what matters most to them. For people in any of these groups, when they request help from mental health services, problems can arise, and some of their core concerns in life may be misunderstood, neglected or pathologised. Key resources which offer potentially positive support for recovery are thereby ignored, sidelined or else become part of the clinical problem rather than its solution.

My Perspective as Author

I am writing as a psychiatrist. I trained in general psychiatry and addictions psychiatry, but most of my clinical work was in the latter subspeciality. For many of my patients, spiritual pathways to recovery were literally life-transforming. For all of my patients who were psychologically and/or physiologically dependent upon substances, fundamental questions arose about whether there was anything that they valued more than the object of their addiction. The salience of addictive patterns of behaviour is such that it tends to erode everything else in life: family, work, morality, identity and self-worth. Recovery depends upon finding something that matters more than the object of addiction. I was therefore always interested to know, 'What matters most to you?' I received many and varied answers to this existential question, mostly not in traditionally religious terms, but for patients in recovery, priorities in life had always had to take a complete change of direction, away from substances and behaviours that were destructive of life and towards the things that gave life.

I am writing not only as a psychiatrist. I am a Christian. I am an honorary chaplain in the Tees, Esk and Wear Valleys NHS Foundation Trust, a priest in the Church of England and an Emeritus Professor in the Institute for Medical Humanities at Durham University. All of these things have shaped my perspectives on psychiatry but also, and perhaps even more, my experiences of illness as a patient and a carer (about which I say more in Chapter 2). I have concluded that spirituality is a core clinical concern for all areas of medicine, not only psychiatry. It is not an 'optional extra' or simply a 'special interest' that is relevant only occasionally. I have reached that conclusion as I have faced illnesses and crises in my own life, and in the lives of those I have loved, as well as in the course of caring for others, pastorally and clinically. Whilst my own narratives have been shaped by my Christian spirituality, I am aware that others use a different vocabulary, and I seek always to be sensitive to this. However, clinicians and clergy often resort to a professional or religious vocabulary which obscures rather than supports processes of personal reflection on suffering. It is important that, as psychiatrists, we are able to present a human face to our patients, and that we do not only act as scientists or technicians.

The Themes of This Book

My contention in this book is that psychiatry is deeply entangled with spirituality, religion and theology. The entanglements of psychiatry with spirituality, theology and faith are far-reaching and influence the views of both clinicians and patients, whether or not they are consciously aware of it. I have therefore illustrated the clinical relevance of these entanglements by the inclusion within each chapter of case studies, engagement with professional practice and examples drawn from experience. I have also addressed the relevant academic literature on spirituality and psychiatry, including – but not only – the scientific evidence base. I want to show that the humanities, especially theology and religious studies, have an important contribution to make. My overall aim, and therefore the central theme of the book, has been to show that spirituality is – whether explicitly acknowledged or not – a core concern of psychiatry, psychiatrists and patients, and thus crucial to patient-centred practice.

The notion of 'entanglement', as used in this book, is obviously metaphorical, seeking to convey a sense of how interrelated and mixed up psychiatry is with spirituality, theology and related disciplines. Perhaps less obviously, as I will explore in Chapter 1, the metaphor derives from research in the critical medical humanities, and I believe that psychiatry needs to engage much more seriously with understandings of the human condition drawn from non-scientific disciplines. The metaphor is employed here in order to show that it is not only undesirable to try to keep the domains of spirituality and psychiatry separate (because this would be to the detriment of patients); it is in fact impossible because they address significantly overlapping concerns. In support of this argument, the book raises some fundamental questions about the nature and practice of psychiatry.

One of the problems with texts on spirituality and psychiatry (including *Spirituality and Psychiatry* – Cook and Powell, 2022) is the tendency to avoid theology almost completely.

This may be justified as being respectful of the theological pluralism amongst readers, clinicians, patients and others. However, the effect of this is to deny theology its disciplinary voice, and to treat specific religious beliefs as unimportant because – implicitly – they are presumed to lack explanatory power. Ironically, avoiding discussion of theology actually assumes and imposes a particular theological stance – the stance of atheism. The approach in the present volume, in contrast, will be to draw on some theological themes of broad relevance across traditions (e.g., image of God, prayer, spirit possession) and, where appropriate, to give specific examples from different faith traditions. It will also emphasise the concept of 'ordinary' theology (Astley and Francis, 2013), especially the theology of patients, as more important in clinical practice than the theologies of academia or religious institutions. What I will not be doing here is to engage in a specifically Christian theology of psychiatry, although I have done that elsewhere (Cook, 2023b).

Religion (as distinct from spirituality) will also be an important theme in this book. I do not share the very negative and superficial view of religion espoused by Thomas Szasz and others. When Szasz suggests that 'man conceives of God in his own image' (Szasz, 1962, p.179), he is making a psychologically valid observation, albeit not a theologically original one. (The idea dates back at least to the work of the German philosopher Ludwig Feuerbach (1804–1872) – Beyers, 2022.) The idea that God 'is a kind of superman', as Szasz asserts (p.179), is a common trope of some strands of atheism, but not one that would be taken seriously by academic theologians. In practice, even in ordinary theology, most images of God are much more complex than this (and will be considered in Chapter 4).

A crucial theme is that of the giving of attention as both a spiritual practice and a clinical skill. As I have explored in Chapter 7, prayer, mindfulness and silence all have a spiritual quality which is fundamentally concerned with attentiveness, and as I reflect back on my own clinical career I think that it has been this quality of attentiveness that has been a central concern of both my spirituality and my professional practice. I have not always been good at it, but I hope I have got better as I have been helped by patients and colleagues to learn to pay attention to the things that matter. However, there are different ways of paying attention, and we all too often revert to a scientific, academic kind of attentiveness which neglects spiritual values. My hope, then, is that psychiatry can become more spiritually attentive, without losing its attentiveness to the sciences of mind and brain. In order to reflect this, I have tried in each chapter to give both a reflective, integrative attention to the relevant clinical and human concerns, as well as an evidence-based and scientific attention to the academic literature.

A final theme is that of the secular, or post-secular, context within which all of these other themes are being considered, at least by readers in the Western world. (I am well aware that for some readers elsewhere in the world the context in which they work will be that not of secularity but of a religious worldview formed by one of the major faith traditions, such as Christianity or Islam. Nonetheless, the global context is still one in which secularism must be addressed as it has been so influential upon the origins and development of the discipline of psychiatry internationally.) Secularity, and its relationship to psychiatry, will be considered especially in Chapters 1 and 8, but will also appear from time to time elsewhere in the book. It has, however, been proposed that we are now entering a post-secular modernity within which religion cannot be ignored, given its historic influences on the values and traditions of supposedly secular societies, its impact upon international politics and its ongoing importance in the lives of 'believing citizens' (Habermas, 2008). Post-secularism has its implications for psychiatry, to which we will return in Chapter 8. However, the whole book is in effect a reflection on what a post-secular psychiatry might look like once its entanglements with religion and spirituality are exposed and acknowledged.

The themes of the book therefore include, centrally, attentiveness to spirituality, its entanglements with psychiatry, and the ordinary theology of patients, all in the context of post-secular modernity. I keep returning to the question of what psychiatry is all about. Whereas Tom Burns (2014) has framed this in terms of a shadow, and Ben Cave (2023) in terms of what we fear most, I increasingly think that it is really about what we desire most, about the light that casts the shadow rather than the shadow itself, even if the shadows have much to teach us about the nature of light. For most of human history, and for most cultures, our deepest desires have usually been expressed in terms of what we now call 'religion' or 'spirituality'. When we experience fear that we may lose hope of attaining these deepest desires, or when we find ourselves in their shadows, we might call on a psychiatrist or on a priest for help, but we hope that they will get us back on track in search of what we most desire. Spiritually attentive psychiatry, as I have called it later in the book, maintains that positive vision of the human quest, whatever vocabulary we may use in trying to articulate it.

The Shape of This Book

This book is intended to be complementary to the second edition of *Spirituality and Psychiatry* (Cook and Powell, 2022), without duplicating the material covered in that volume. It draws on topics and examples which were either not covered in that volume or else only addressed there in passing. These include the importance of engagement with the critical medical humanities (especially theology and the study of spirituality), the spirituality of the psychiatrist, the hearing of spiritually significant voices, and demon possession. However, the intention in doing this has not been merely to fill in the gaps left by *Spirituality and Psychiatry*, but rather to paint a picture of how spirituality and psychiatry are interrelated. It is a completely different kind of book. The shape of this book is therefore not constructed around either the diagnostic categories of psychiatry or its subspeciality interests.

Because this book is a single-author work, unlike *Spirituality and Psychiatry*, I have been able to paint a picture of psychiatry as I see it. This is a more personal, integrated and (I hope) creative perspective, pushing some of the boundaries. My portrait of psychiatry will, I expect, be controversial in places and will not necessarily reflect a likeness that all psychiatrists will recognise. However, I believe that it is also completely in accord with the holistic model of psychiatry presented within the *Silver Guide* to the revised curricula of the Royal College of Psychiatrists (RCPsych, 2022). What I am presenting here is a personal vision of how that holistic model of psychiatry might look in practice. Whilst I am questioning the assumptions that we make about spirituality in psychiatry, and proposing different ways of seeing and doing things, this is ultimately about seeking a holistic, patient-centred understanding of psychiatry in its wider human context. As such, I hope that it will be recognisable for psychiatrists and patients of all faiths or none. Where there is dissent, I hope that it will generate constructive discussion.

In order to paint this person-centred picture of psychiatry, and after exploring some of the core themes of the book in more depth in Chapter 1, I turn in Chapter 2 to the spirituality of the psychiatrist. This may seem an odd way to go about painting a picture in which I see patients as central, but I don't think we can understand our patients properly if we are not first and last able to be self-reflective about the way in which we handle our own spirituality, as human beings and as a profession. It is thus only in Chapter 3 that I get to the heart of what I think patient-centred spirituality is really all about.

In Chapter 4 I turn to the complex interdisciplinary relationship between the science of psychiatry and theology. I think that one of the reasons that we struggle to see the importance of spirituality to psychiatry is that (at least in the Western world) we have lost sight of the ways in which the European Enlightenment has distorted our understanding of the formal academic engagement between science and theology. Even more importantly, we have lost sight of the ways in which 'ordinary' theology affects the thinking of patients about their faith and their illness. In order to illustrate the importance of this, I have again had to be selective, and I have chosen the important topic of God image as illustrative of the wider concerns of what I am calling here 'clinical theology'.

Chapters 5 and 6 are, respectively, about psychiatric phenomenology and spiritual struggles. Because each of these topics really deserves a book all to itself, I have chosen specific examples to illustrate the broader themes. Chapter 5 is therefore based on my work on auditory verbal hallucinations (and especially spiritually significant voices), and Chapter 6 is based on a case study of a patient who believed that he was possessed by evil spirits. So much more could be written about entanglements of spirituality with other aspects of psychiatric phenomenology than hallucinations, and possession states are only one of many kinds of spiritual struggle. Nonetheless, I hope that they illustrate some of the broader themes to which I am trying to draw attention in this book. Spirituality is intimately interwoven with psychiatric phenomenology, whether implicitly or explicitly, and spiritual struggles of diverse kinds become entangled with mental illness in a complex, bidirectional interrelationship.

Clinical psychiatry is all about finding ways to bring healing and to facilitate processes of recovery. In Chapter 7 I have therefore turned to spiritual interventions, or treatments. I have again tried to focus on some of the topics which I think have been neglected, in this case the question of giving careful attention in psychiatry, and the importance of silence as both a spiritual and a psychological practice. However, I have also addressed here the controversial topic of prayer and the much-discussed employment of mindfulness as a spiritual treatment in psychiatry. Patients want to know that we are giving them our careful attention, and there is a spiritual dimension to this careful attentiveness which may be helpfully (or unhelpfully) expressed in prayer, mindfulness and silence. I am proposing a spiritually attentive and patient-centred approach to psychiatry, within which prayer, mindfulness and silence each have their proper place.

Finally, in Chapter 8, I consider the ways in which psychiatrists manage spirituality professionally, especially in relation to boundaries. When it comes to affirming the import-ance of spirituality in psychiatry, boundaries have so often been seen as the problem, whereas in fact I see them as the solution. Psychiatry is – or should be – concerned with creating safe clinical spaces within which positive spiritual and psychological transform-ation can take place. These safe spaces are paradoxically less, not more, easily created in a secular society than in a religious one. However, in the post-secular age that we are now entering, we need to look again at the boundaries that create and protect these safe therapeutic spaces. The important boundaries are often seen as being professional and social, whereas I believe that they are primarily inner and psychological. They are also not there as natural features, dividing the landscape like walls or fences; rather, they are clinically created with the purpose of integration. Whilst this may sound paradoxical and somewhat counter-intuitive, I hope that the picture will nonetheless become clear in this final chapter.

The shape of this book is therefore not moulded by psychiatric taxonomies, by neuroscience or by any of the other chapter headings of traditional psychiatric textbooks; rather, it is formed by the spiritual challenges facing patients and their psychiatrists in clinical context, their phenomenology, their boundaries and their entanglements.

Psychiatrists

I want to make clear at the outset that I am not in any way suggesting that atheist or agnostic psychiatrists are not as good at attending to spiritual concerns in clinical practice, compared with their religious colleagues. Nor am I writing only for those who consider themselves to be either spiritual or religious (or both). I have huge regard for the clinical and spiritual sensitivities of many who do not share my Christian worldview. There is no 'view from nowhere' and we all approach our clinical and academic work from a particular, situated and personal viewpoint. Over the years, I have personally received more complaints from patients about proselytising by atheist and agnostic psychiatrists than I have about proselytising for particular spiritual or religious beliefs. However, there are atheist psychiatrists who are very sensitive to the spiritual concerns of their patients, and there are religious psychiatrists who are very insensitive.

We are all prone to slip into our own comfortable ways of viewing things, and to imagine that others would be better off if they viewed things as we do. I have often been approached by Christians saying that they would like to see a Christian psychiatrist (one example of which is given in Chapter 3) and I almost always say that they need to see a good psychiatrist, not necessarily a Christian one. I believe that what is needed is spiritually attentive clinical care, and that this can be provided by any good psychiatrist, regardless of his or her spiritual/religious beliefs, or lack of them. So, my core message in this book is that psychiatrists, whoever they may be, need to keep spirituality in mind, and that this is central to a person-centred, holistic understanding of what psychiatry is all about.

Readers of This Book

As I write this book, my main intended audience is psychiatrists, both trainees and consultants. However, I hope that the book will have wider appeal amongst all who are concerned about mental health, the allied mental health professions, especially mental health chaplains, and patients who want to reflect critically on their experiences of mental illness and psychiatric care. I'm hoping that the book will facilitate reflection on clinical work, provoke debate within the field and encourage creative and critical thinking about the relationship of spirituality to the biopsychosocial model in a pluralistic and global psychiatric environment.

Vocabulary

A few words may be in order with regard to vocabulary. As was the case when I was editing *Spirituality and Psychiatry* (Cook, 2022c, p.xxii), I have chosen to use the word 'patient' to refer to those who experience mental illness and seek help from psychiatrists. This word generally seems to be preferred by patients themselves, although, unsurprisingly, there are those who prefer other terms, such as 'service users' or 'experts by experience'. I prefer 'patient' because I am a patient (as well as a doctor) myself, albeit not a psychiatric patient, and the tendency to avoid the term in our particular area of medicine seems to me to express a subtle form of stigma against mental illness. The word 'patient' also has etymological connections with a spiritual virtue of patience, which is consonant with the positive message of spirituality that I wish to convey in the book. For similar reasons, I will use terminology of mental illness or mental disorder rather than the euphemisms which seek to avoid implication of a medical model. All of this is in support of a vision of patient-centred medicine in which patients are people, and in which doctors and patients share a common humanity in which we all face our own experiences of illness and suffering in body, mind and spirit.

As I hope may already be clear, when I employ the word 'theology' I am including atheism and agnosticism as theological perspectives which need to be taken seriously. I therefore have a very broad view of what constitutes theology, within which one view is that there is no God, a view that we might refer to as 'atheology'. Similarly, spirituality encompasses a wide range of worldviews including atheistic spiritualities, those who identify as SBNR and the spiritualities associated with the world's major religions. To some extent, then, it is worldviews that I am concerned with, in a broad sense: 'A worldview is a collection of attitudes, values, stories and expectations about the world around us, which inform our every thought and action' (Gray, 2011, p.58). Worldviews do not only derive from spirituality and religion, but it is the spiritual and theological aspects of worldviews that I will be most concerned with in this book, in relation to psychiatry.

Case Studies

Finally, a word of explanation is in order in regard to the clinical material presented in this book. I have employed various strategies in order to ensure that cases cannot be recognised. This has included changing identifying details and amalgamating different cases into one. Some of the stories relate to patients whom I saw many decades ago. However, some issues are seemingly universal. In a public lecture that I gave a few years ago, I invented an entirely imaginary case study in order to illustrate some of the issues that arise in relation to religious faith and depression. I told a story of a completely fictional patient, whom I called Agnes. A woman whom I had never met before came forward after the lecture and said, 'I am Agnes!' It is therefore entirely likely that some readers may recognise themselves, or people whom they know, in the clinical examples that I have given in this book, but this will only be because the issues concerned have wide currency and are far from unusual.

With hindsight, I wish that I had kept better records of my clinical encounters over the years. Ben Cave's book, cited in my opening paragraph, is an excellent example of how helpful this can be. I'd like to go back and review in detail how my attitudes have changed and to reflect again on clinical encounters earlier in my career in the light of what I have learnt in the years that have followed. However, the memories that endure are the lessons that my patients taught me about suffering, spirituality and how to be a better psychiatrist. Also enduring are the important clinical lessons that I learnt from my consultants when I was a trainee, and later from my clinical colleagues in my peer group, and in the Spirituality and Psychiatry Special Interest Group (SPSIG) at the Royal College of Psychiatrists. These were usually not about things that you get asked about in membership examinations for the RCPsych, but they are about things that make the difference between being merely an adequate psychiatrist and a really good one. They were about compassion, humanity, wisdom and spiritual attentiveness. Even if there are shadows in psychiatry, there is also a lot of light.

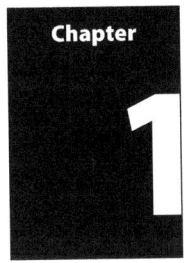

Entanglements of Psychiatry with Spirituality

Looking back, Jenny thinks that her symptoms began when she was only 12 years old, but receiving a diagnosis of obsessional compulsive disorder was still a shock when it came in her early twenties. I first met her not in my work as a psychiatrist but in my role as an honorary NHS chaplain, by which time she was training to be a chef. Her obsessional thoughts about sharp knives and contamination of food had begun to cause problems for her at work. She had distressing mental images of harm that she might cause herself or others. A GP (primary care physician) had referred her for psychiatric assessment.

Jenny was preoccupied with fears of death. When babysitting as a teenager she had had worries that the infant she was caring for would stop breathing, and so would be constantly checking that the child was still okay. If she knew someone was going to die, she reasoned, she would want to tell them that she loved them. Extrapolating from this, in a form of thought-action fusion (TAF) (Shafran and Rachman, 2004), she worried that if she did tell her family or boyfriend that she loved them then they might actually die. This, in turn, made it difficult for her to tell them that she loved them.

A consultant psychiatrist diagnosed obsessive-compulsive disorder (OCD), started Jenny on citalopram, and referred her for psychotherapy. The therapist began a programme of exposure and response prevention. She made good progress on treatment, but still struggled to manage aspects of her condition which, she felt, neither the GP nor the psychiatrist had fully understood.

Jenny is a Christian, a member of the congregation of her local parish church where charismatic spirituality involves expressive acts such as raising hands in praise to God when singing contemporary worship songs. Biblical teaching in the church emphasises spontaneity in prayer and obedience to the Holy Spirit. Jenny found herself distracted during church worship by intrusive thoughts about whether or not it was the Holy Spirit that was prompting her to raise her hands. She didn't want to be disobedient to God, or to miss out on opportunities to draw close to him, but how could she know if this was God or not?

At night, Jenny experienced 'promptings' to get out of bed and pray, so that she was losing sleep and getting increasingly tired during the day. She feared that – if she did not pray as she should – she might not be forgiven for wrong things she had done during the past day, or that she might die in her sleep and go to hell. She feared that if she had not prayed for her loved ones, bad things might happen to them, or they might die. She feared not being thankful to God for all the good things in her life. This had been made worse by a minister in the church who used to ask, 'What would you have tomorrow if you only had what you thanked God for today?' She also felt anxiety if she missed her prayers before bedtime, which consequently made these devotions an obligation rather than a joy and further enhanced her tiredness. There was thus a lot of fear and anxiety, and it revolved mainly around Jenny's Christian spirituality.

A Sunday sermon in church, just after Christmas, had focussed on the story of the 'slaughter of the innocents' (Matthew 2:16–18), a rather gruesome biblical story in which King Herod murdered thousands of innocent children. This left Jenny with particularly distressing and intrusive mental images of murdered children. She became angry with God that he would allow all of this to happen to her and frustrated that her illness was affecting all the areas of her life that were most important to her. In her conversation with me, she voiced the question: 'Is nothing sacred?' She was finding it difficult to disentangle her faith from her illness.

Jenny had told her psychiatrist about these concerns but, although he seemed to understand at one level, he clearly didn't appreciate why the spiritual aspects of her illness were so important to her. The psychotherapist had been a little more understanding and had incorporated some of the religious compulsions into her programme of exposure and response prevention. However, Jenny found that medical professionals generally didn't seem to understand her faith, or the particular distress that she experienced because of the way that her illness was disrupting her spiritual life and causing her to question everything. She was even more worried about what folks at church would think about her illness. The failure of medical professionals to understand the importance of Jenny's faith led to omission of significant aspects of her illness from treatment planning. The lack of understanding of members of her faith community in relation to mental health issues left her not knowing where to go with the important, and very valid, spiritual and theological questions that she had about what she was experiencing.

In our conversations together, Jenny and I were able to explore illness in the context of faith and faith in the context of illness, so that she was able to find a way of integrating the different areas of her life with her Christian worldview. Illness in the context of faith was hard to accept. Why would God allow this to happen? Looking back, Jenny realises that – as a result of her illness – her faith had become very rule-bound and obligational. As she put it, she had lost sight of the grace of God. Faith in the context of illness was more complicated than she felt it should be. Now, however, as she enters into a phase of recovery where she is able to get back to work and enjoy life again, she is able to be more discerning about inner 'promptings' and where they come from, spiritually speaking. This has made faith a bit more complex but has also deepened her awareness of the importance and nature of her relationship with God. She has learnt to be more discerning about the inner promptings that she experiences, and to distinguish more easily between what she believes is the voice of the Holy Spirit and what is more obviously obsessional. Her faith and her self-awareness have deepened as a result, all of which has enhanced and promoted her recovery from her mental health condition.

Reflecting with Jenny

Reflecting on Jenny's illness, I'm sure that all psychiatrists will easily identify the features of an obsessive-compulsive disorder. The recurring, intrusive thoughts and mental images that she experienced are a very typical example of the psychopathology of this condition, although, actually, intrusive thoughts are experienced by almost everyone in the wider population in a sub-clinical, and less distressing, form (Clark et al., 2014). The themes of concern around sharp objects and food contamination are common ones. Compulsive checking is similarly characteristic, albeit this was a less distressing feature of the illness as far as Jenny was concerned. I don't think that the diagnosis was in much doubt, and the treatment prescribed was reassuringly and rapidly effective. An observant psychiatrist, as indeed her clinician was, would have noticed that the spiritual 'promptings' also had an obsessional character. However, reflecting *on* this aspect of her illness, as merely another instance of psychopathology, risks an important omission that could have been avoided by reflecting *with* Jenny on her spiritual experience.

The phenomenology of Jenny's story is both an account of an illness and an account of a spiritual experience (or series of experiences) in the context of Christian faith. It is understandable, although not necessarily excusable, that mental health professionals should focus more on the illness than on the spiritual experiences. A person-centred account might more readily identify spiritual concerns as the primary feature of the story, in support of which psychiatry has something important to offer by way of a diagnosis that supports a treatment plan which, in turn, leads to relief of distress. However, the treatment plan is inadequate if it leaves the salient area of the patient's concerns unaddressed. How is Jenny to make sense of the confusion she experiences in relation to distinguishing between prompt-ings of the Holy Spirit and obsessional anxieties due to her illness? The spiritual aspects of Jenny's illness were not a peripheral matter, and they were not adequately addressed by clinicians who, at best, treated them as part of the illness or, at worst, ignored them. Equally, members of her local church did not know how to help her with her illness and, such was the stigma, she did not feel able to talk to most of them about it.

Reflecting with Jenny, and seeing things from her perspective, the phenomenology of spiritual experience and that of psychopathology were all mixed up with each other. This was a central concern, raising questions about how to deal with an illness in the context of faith, and how to address spiritual concerns in the context of an illness. Just dealing with the illness was, at best, addressing only half of the problem, and the less important half at that. We might speculate that, in the mind of her psychiatrist, faith was not his problem, or else was only peripheral. Actually, that is a kind of mix-up too – mixing up a personal pragmatic atheism[1] with a professional role as clinician and thereby failing to see things from Jenny's spiritual perspective. Similarly, we might speculate that folks at church would view Jenny's illness as a failure of her faith in some way, perhaps as something that wouldn't have happened if she had had more faith, or – even worse – not an illness at all but a failure to be obedient to the promptings of the Holy Spirit. Again, this seems to be a mix-up on their part, a mixing up of illness and faith in such a way as to obscure almost completely the role of the former in giving rise to her distress.

These mix-ups, or entanglements, of spirituality and mental illness also betray stigma and prejudice on the part of those concerned. Clinicians, whether they consciously mean to or not, easily convey a largely subliminal message that they don't want to talk about spirituality (which, in their minds, may be only a part of the illness anyway), and members

---

[1] Pragmatic atheism, in a secular society, assumes that the world 'may be understood in its own terms, without immediate or explicit reference to God' (McFadyen, 2000, p.6). It thus 'assumes the practical irrelevance of God's existence to the disciplines of reflection and practice we all use as we interpret and act in the world' (p.7) and expects public discourse to be conducted without reference to God. In drawing everyone into utilising such frameworks of understanding, it requires of them a performance of atheism, albeit not a conscious or explicit declaration of atheistic belief (McFadyen, 2000, pp.6–11).

of a faith community easily convey a similarly implicit message that faithful Christians (or Muslims, or Jews, or others) shouldn't experience mental illness. This leaves the patient – the person – at the centre of all of this in a position of not being properly understood by anyone and being stigmatised by everyone. It is a lonely place to be.

Entanglements

Entanglement has become a focus of interest in a range of different literatures in recent years, from physics to sociology (Fitzgerald and Callard, 2016). In the critical medical humanities, it has raised important questions about the ways in which different disciplines and professions engage with each other as they seek to understand, and treat, the human condition. This is not a question of trying to disentangle complex phenomena; it is rather an active seeking out of entanglement as a better way of understanding things:

> What holds together much of the research employing the concept of 'entanglement' is an intuition that some set of things, commonly held to be separate from one another (indeed, that define themselves precisely with reference to their separability) – science and justice, humans and non-humans, settlers and natives – not only might have something in common, but also, in fact, may be quite *inseparable* from one another. (Fitzgerald and Callard, 2016, p.39)

My contention in this book is that spirituality and religion are inherently entangled with psychiatry. Boundaries and differences do matter, as will be discussed later in the book, but these are things that are necessarily created, and should not be seen as things that have to be overcome in order to achieve an integrative perspective (Fitzgerald and Callard, 2016, p.41). Rather, spirituality and religion exist in a fluid, relational and dynamic entanglement with psychiatry which offers scope for a different way of seeing things than the one that currently fuels the oppositional boundary disputes that will be discussed in Chapter 8.

Just as academic and professional disciplines are entangled, so are people. In anthropology, a distinction is made between the 'dividual' and the individual self. Whereas the individual self, so highly prized in individualistic Western society, is understood as a discrete entity, the dividual self is both more fragmented and more integrated:

> In the simplest terms, the individual is considered to be an indivisible self or person. That is, it refers to something like the essential core, or spirit of a singular human being, which as a whole, defines that self in its particularity . . . .. By contrast, the dividual is considered to be divisible, comprising a complex of separable – interrelated but essentially independent – dimensions or aspects. The individual is thus monadic, while the dividual is fractal; the individual is atomistic, while the dividual is always socially embedded; the individual is an autonomous social actor, the author of his or her own actions, while the dividual is a heteronomous actor performing a culturally written script; the individual is a free agent, while the dividual is determined by cultural structures; the individual is egocentric, and the dividual is sociocentric. (Smith, 2012, p.53)

If the concept is related to self (rather than person), the dividual self 'according to modern psychiatry' shows signs of severe psychopathology (Spiro, 1993, p.109). However, the concept arguably relates more to the person, rather than the self, and as such is less concerned with psychology or psychiatry and more with sociology and anthropology. In any case the distinction between the dividual and the individual, arising originally from comparisons of Western and non-Western concepts of self/person, has been increasingly recognised as representing contrasting modes of personhood that all human beings inhabit. It is less concerned with distinctions between people, Western and non-Western, and more with different ways of seeing ourselves in the world.

In *A Secular Age*, Charles Taylor (2007) contrasts what he calls the 'porous' self of an enchanted premodern world and the 'buffered' self of the modern disenchanted world. The buffered self experiences a much stronger sense of the boundary between the self and the world (including others), whereas the porous self has more permeable boundaries and sees greater connectedness both with other human beings and with a wider order of material and spiritual things. As Karl Smith (2012) has pointed out, the porous self and the dividual self share some significant things in common, albeit the distinctions in relation to the former have been based more on changes in worldview associated with European history, and the latter more upon cross-cultural comparisons. Smith suggests that the human subject is inherently porous and that this is actually a good thing:

> The sense of porousness, the porosity that I want to advance here, is not an openness to spirits and causal powers. Rather I am attempting to invoke the ways in which the human subject is a thoroughly permeated being – one that is permeated by social others; by socially ascribed meanings, roles, norms and mores – while also remaining open to 'nature', the 'world' and the mysteries of existence. I am positing a sense of the human person who has inner depths, as per the Freudian psyche, but without the rigid inner/outer distinction inherited from Cartesian philosophy. (Smith, 2012, p.60)

Whilst I accept Smith's point completely in the context of his argument, Taylor's articulation of the concept of porosity clearly does include an openness to a spiritual world, as well as to a social and natural one. The porous self, in many ways like the dividual self, is radically entangled with a wider natural, sociocultural and spiritual order. The buffered self, so characteristic of our secular age, seeks to deny this, but is that a good thing to do?

Spirituality

So much metaphorical ink has been spilt in an attempt to 'define' spirituality that it easily completely obscures the key issues in relation to psychiatry. Spirituality is an inherently complex and contested concept which eludes simple definition. It is virtually impossible to distinguish from psychological outcome variables in research, so that Harold Koenig (one of the leading scientific researchers in this field today) has argued that, in terms of research methodology, it is better to study religion or religiosity (Koenig, 2008a). However, as Koenig acknowledges, spirituality is still a useful term in clinical practice. It allows a more inclusive conversation than does, for example, the concept of religion. To this end, some years ago now, I proposed the following definition, which has subsequently been used in the position statement on spirituality and psychiatry adopted by the Royal College of Psychiatrists (RCPsych):

> Spirituality is a distinctive, potentially creative and universal dimension of human experience arising both within the inner subjective awareness of individuals and within communities, social groups and traditions. It may be experienced as relationship with that which is intimately 'inner', immanent and personal, within the self and others, and/or as relationship with that which is wholly 'other', transcendent and beyond the self. It is experienced as being

of fundamental or ultimate importance and is thus concerned with matters of meaning and purpose in life, truth and values. (Cook, 2004, pp.548–549)

This definition is not perfect; it is prolix, and some significant work has been done by others over the last two decades in terms of further clarifying the different components of the concept which might be important in clinical practice (e.g., De Brito Sena et al., 2021). However, it is inclusive of those who are spiritual but not religious (SBNR) as well as those who adopt religious forms of spiritualty, which was one of the original objectives in developing it. It incorporates some of the key concerns – relationality, transcendence, meaning – without requiring subscription to any of the more divisive stances in debates over theology, religion or tradition. It was intended to open up a constructive conversation, rather than promote defensive arguments, and I think that it has helped towards this end. However, like all definitions of spirituality, it indirectly implies that scientists might study it as a 'thing' that is amenable to objective investigation, and this is somewhat in contradiction to its highly subjective nature. If it is truly concerned with transcendence, this may simply not be possible in any meaningful way, given that science is concerned with the immanent order of things. If it is possible at all, then it will involve studying proxy variables (such as meaning and purpose in life, or religious identity) which will always move the conversation to a slightly different field of meaning than that of 'spirituality'.

Perhaps it is important here, in passing, to note some of the things that spirituality is not. It is not a proxy for religion (which will be discussed later), albeit there is a significant overlap and connection between the two topics. For some people, spirituality and religion are almost opposites; for others, they are almost co-terminous. It is not a shorthand for some kind of dualism of supernatural and material domains, even if some people do see it in exactly this way. By the same token, it does not mean 'belief in God'. In many ways, it is easier to say what spirituality is not than to say what it is.

The concept of spirituality is inherently problematic. For example, I know that some of my colleagues see it as unhelpful in relation to boundary issues (which I will discuss further in Chapter 8). However, that does not necessarily mean that we should dispense with it; rather – I believe – we should engage with it in a critical and thoughtful way. My major concern here is the way in which it is seen as an optional extra, rather than as a core concern of the biopsychosocial model which has been so central to psychiatry for the last several decades. Ironically, it is many of those who share my concerns with the importance of spirituality with whom I differ here. A common trope has been to propose the expansion of the biopsychosocial model to become a biopsychosocial-spiritual model (e.g., Kuhn, 1988; McKee and Chappel, 1992; Galbadage et al., 2020). This fundamentally fails to take into account the entanglement of spirituality with the biopsychosocial domains and simply makes it easier to say that the latter are the responsibility of health professionals, whilst the former is the responsibility of clergy, chaplains and spiritual care professionals.

Spirituality is radically, and inextricably, entangled with the biopsychosocial concerns of psychiatry. Starting with the biology, George Vaillant (2013), for example, has suggested that what we 'really' mean by spirituality is a constellation of eight emotions – 'awe, love/ attachment, trust/faith, compassion, gratitude, forgiveness, joy and hope' (p.590) – that have historically been neglected by psychiatry. Spirituality is, he believes, 'not about ideas, sacred texts and theology' (p.590) but, rather, 'all about emotion and social connection' (p.590) which, in turn, he observes, are dependent on the limbic system rather than the cortex. '[R]eligion arises from cognitive culture; spirituality arises from limbic biology' (p.592). To take a rather different example, transliminality, a rather broad concept, thought by Thalbourne and Maltby (2008) to be associated with mystical and paranormal experiences (amongst other things), is said to be associated with temporal lobe lability. Yet another example may be found in the attentional concerns of spirituality (discussed in Chapter 7), which relate to biologically based specialisation of the different modes of attention made possible by circuits in the left and right hemispheres of the brain. Indeed, however spirituality might be interpreted, there has to be some biological basis for it in neuroscience unless, of course, one adopts a completely dualistic model of anthropology with all its concomitant Cartesian problems.

Spirituality is further entangled, as Koenig (2008a) has cogently observed, with human psychology; so much so that it is virtually impossible to operationalise it in empirical research in non-psychological terms. Measures of spiritual well-being typically include such things as 'optimism, forgiveness, gratitude, meaning and purpose in life, peacefulness, harmony, and general wellbeing' (Koenig, 2008a, p.349), all of which are also aspects of mental health, and primarily psychological variables. Ralph Piedmont (1999) has proposed that spirituality, understood as a motivational domain of 'spiritual transcendence', actually represents a sixth factor of personality, alongside those included in the now well-established five-factor model. None of this should be surprising. Spirituality may be centrally concerned with transcendence, but transcendence is a concept with which people engage in cognitive and emotional ways. Even if spiritual experiences are sometimes ineffable, they are still psychologically mediated and they have cognitive and affective concomitants. Even theological virtues such as hope are inextricably entangled with psychological states of well-being (Espedal, 2021).

Finally, and equally unsurprisingly, spirituality is concerned with social and cultural dimensions of well-being. Whilst spirituality is often portrayed as subjective, and individually orientated, in contrast to the social structures of religion, it is also usually defined as relational. It is centrally concerned with relationships with self, with others, and with some wider or transcendent reality, variously defined (e.g., Cook, 2004). Spiritualities that are religious in a traditional sense even more obviously include a social and cultural dimension in that religion (as discussed later) necessarily involves shared systems of symbolism, ritual and meaning.

None of these biopsychosocial entanglements, however, completely captures what spirituality is all about, and it cannot satisfactorily be reduced to any of them. In a similar way, much can be said about experiences of falling in love, as they affect us socially, emotionally and physiologically, but none of these scientific accounts adequately conveys the human experience in all its fullness. Spirituality is elusive, but it is more adequately conveyed by disciplines historically considered to be the humanities than it is by those considered to be sciences. Often experienced as ineffable, it can sometimes be more effectively portrayed in art than in words. Even within the disciplines of theology and the (academic) study of spirituality, it is often better portrayed as apophatic, in terms of unknowing or not knowing, than it is in terms of what can positively be said. It evokes a heartfelt search for whatever is held to be most deeply important and desirable, and yet it always hints at something more, something not entirely within the human grasp.

A patient-centred approach to Jenny's distress reveals that spirituality was deeply important to her, both in terms of her wider enjoyment of life and in terms of understanding the nature of her distress. A corresponding treatment plan was needed to address the biological, psychological and social dimensions of this spirituality. Because spirituality was not understood as integrally entangled with all of these dimensions of well-being, the treatment plan that was offered failed to address some of her central concerns. Because the professional vision of recovery was conceived of in reductively biopsychosocial terms, it failed to grasp a vision of 'something more'. It failed to convey empathy for the things that were most important to Jenny; it failed to appreciate the things that she loved; it failed to keep spirituality in mind.

Religion

No less metaphorical ink has been spilt in attempts to define the concept of religion than in attempts to define spirituality. Ultimately, religion is a concept whose 'meaning is unstable and contested, and . . . cannot be defined so as to specify anything uniquely' (Taves, 2011, p.58), but precise conceptual definitions are not necessarily what is needed in relation to research or clinical practice in psychiatry.

Amongst the many definitions of religion that have been proposed, that offered by Clifford Geertz has been amongst the most influential: '(1) a system of symbols which acts to (2) establish powerful, pervasive, and long-lasting moods and motivations in men by (3) formulating conceptions of a general order of existence and (4) clothing these conceptions with such an aura of factuality that (5) the moods and motivations seem uniquely realistic' (Geertz, 1993, p.90). It might be argued that this definition is too broad, and it may draw in things that we would not normally consider religious. It may also not say enough (at least directly) about some things that are really important to many religious people. However, it does draw attention to some of the concerns that are important in relation to psychiatry. Religion is concerned with symbols that evoke affective and motivational change and provide existential meaning. There were important symbols within the phenomenology and narrative of Jenny's story, notably her reference to the sacred, that provide clues to the way in which her illness and faith were entangled. Her Christian faith offered an important resource for positive religious coping – in terms of emotional regulation and the search for existential meaning – which was almost completely neglected by her clinicians.

In her 'building blocks' approach to religion, Ann Taves (2011) looks at the ways in which religion involves a setting apart of 'special things'. The special things that provide the building blocks that Taves identifies within this framework include anomalous experiences of agency, anomalous places, objects, experiences and events (without agency), and ideal things. Amongst the ideal things (we might better, here, call them 'themes') identified by Taves that make a significant appearance, implicitly or explicitly, in Jenny's psychopathology are: transcendence, reality, truth, good, evil, purity and perfection. The setting for these ideal things was in some special/spiritual places and events, including worship in church and liminal places between life and death, arising as a result of TAF, in relation to those whom she loved, or for whom she had responsibility. The central concern for Jenny, however, was with anomalous experiences of agency, that is, the inner 'promptings' which she experienced as being from God and yet which, because of her illness, she doubted and questioned. In a very real sense, Jenny's illness struck to the heart of her identity and experience as a Christian. As she succinctly and rhetorically summarised in her own words, 'Is nothing sacred?'

Like spirituality, religion is deeply entangled with the biopsychosocial matrix that is the central concern of psychiatry (see, for example, Argyle, 2002; Rim et al., 2019).

The Person-Centred Holistic Model of Psychiatry

The RCPsych *Silver Guide* (2022), which sets out to help new trainees (and their trainers) navigate professional formation in psychiatry, offers a list of foundational concepts which underpin good professional practice. The vision of psychiatry that it presents includes an understanding of the patient as a whole person, 'body, mind and spirit', and 'a model of the person which draws on the social sciences, neurosciences and the humanities' (p.6). It urges its readers to take into account the 'impact of culture, religion and social systems on individuals' and encourages them to adopt 'a compassionate clinical approach, based on both values and evidence'. It highlights the importance of 'a holistic person-centred care approach for patients, taking into account physical, psychological and spiritual needs' (p.6).

This holistic approach to psychiatry is inspiring, but how is it to be realised? Few psychiatrists have a grounding in the humanities, and postgraduate training in psychiatry usually offers very little on spirituality or religion (and nothing on theology) to complement a highly scientific curriculum in which the biopsychosocial aspects of psychiatry are otherwise addressed in depth. Candidates for the membership examination of the RCPsych might be forgiven for thinking that, in reality, the biological, psychological and social elements of the whole person are important, but spirituality is not.

The *Silver Guide* is, of course, not the whole story. The spiritual needs of patients do appear in the RCPsych curriculum documents, albeit alongside a heavy weighting towards an understanding of the biopsychosocial that omits discussion of spirituality. The College has a helpful position statement, *Recommendations on Spirituality and Religion for Psychiatrists*, in which guidance is provided for assessment, clinical practice, training and collaborative working (Royal College of Psychiatrists, 2013). Spiritual and religious concerns are integral to the recovery approach, which is now central to psychiatric practice (Leamy et al., 2011), and are further affirmed in a report of the Person-Centred Training and Curriculum (PCTC) Scoping Group (2018). A number of other College publications address the topic, including, notably, *Spirituality and Psychiatry* (Cook and Powell, 2022). However, there have also been sometimes heated debates around such things as professional boundaries, such that many trainees (not to mention consultants) feel uncertain about how to address spirituality/religion in actual clinical practice (Cook, 2013a). The Spirituality and Psychiatry Special Interest Group (SPSIG) at the RCPsych has, for over 25 years, offered continuing professional development for psychiatrists on spirituality/religion, including day conferences and webinars, as well as an online CPD module (RCPsych, 2024). As will be discussed further in Chapter 8, psychiatrists in other countries around the world have pursued a similar agenda in relation to research, teaching and clinical practice, nationally and internationally.

Outside the circles of groups such as the SPSIG of the RCPsych, or the Caucus on Religion and Spirituality of the American Psychiatric Association, it is not clear how many psychiatrists see spirituality/religion as central to their daily work. Awareness of the importance of these issues is undoubtedly much greater than it was over a quarter of a century ago, when SPSIG was founded, and attendance at webinars and training events (such as those offered by SPSIG) suggests that there is a widespread interest in the topic. This book is offered partly in response to that demand but also with the intention of provoking greater interest and debate amongst those psychiatrists who remain to be convinced of the importance of the topic for their daily work. For these, and for other interested readers, what are the currently available options for integrating spirituality/religion more fully into clinical practice and research in psychiatry?

From Biopsychosocial Model to Patient-Centred Care

The simplest way in which to envisage change is to acknowledge that the biopsychosocial model, on its own, does not go far enough. Spirituality therefore needs to be added as a fourth dimension, so as to create a biopsychosocial-spiritual model (Kuhn, 1988). This certainly gives visibility to the topic (or, at least, it would if widely adopted) but it also suggests that spirituality is an 'add-on' and therefore, potentially, something that can be neglected wherever psychiatrists see the biological, psychological and sociocultural aspects of well-being as their primary concern. Even more importantly, as discussed earlier, it fails to recognise that spirituality is in fact an inextricably entangled concern of the three biopsychosocial domains. It is simply not possible to employ the biopsychosocial model properly without addressing the spiritual within the biological, the psychological and the social, even though this is in fact exactly what many psychiatrists try to do every day.

Another approach would be to recognise that spiritual/religious concerns are already identified as important elements within, for example, the recovery approach, transcultural psychiatry and patient-centred care, and that nothing new is needed so much as to ensure that it is not neglected within teaching, research and practice in these areas. The need, then, is to improve quality and practice of care according to existing models, rather than to see the need for anything new. As with the earlier comments on the biopsychosocial model, there is much to commend this approach, except for the invisibility of spirituality/religion within it. The danger is that it is not prioritised unless or until it is explicitly mentioned. Given that many patients are already hesitant to mention the topic, there is every likelihood that it will not be mentioned and that it will constantly be forgotten.

Taking a more radical line, others have suggested that what is really needed is a complete 'paradigm shift'. This is well illustrated by one of the founding members of SPSIG, Larry Culliford (2011b), in his book *The Psychology of Spirituality*. The idea of paradigm shift was introduced in the natural sciences by Thomas Kuhn in the 1960s but has since been applied in many other contexts. As summarised by Culliford: 'A paradigm shift involves a major conceptual change in both theory and practice. It is necessarily a development or extension of what has gone before' (Culliford, 2011b, p.91). Culliford sees such a shift taking place in relation to spirituality in Western society: 'Western culture is undergoing a significant paradigm shift – from a materialist view, based on the assumptions of dualism, rationalism, positivism and empiricism, towards a naturalistic understanding that acknowledges the significance of such things as personal stories, emotions and experiences that cannot be explained purely in terms of science' (Culliford, 2002, p.250). More particularly, he sees this shift taking place within psychiatry and the allied disciplines: 'The psycho-spiritual paradigm involves recognition that spirituality involves a universal yet deeply personal and essentially subjective dimension of human experience, about which it can be hard to communicate in words' (Culliford, 2011a, p.46). I largely agree with Culliford, but I'm not seeing a recognition of the need for such a paradigm shift amongst the majority of my professional colleagues. There is also a problem with positing the universality of spirituality. Some people consistently identify as neither spiritual nor religious. Whilst I may have conversations with them, as colleagues and patients, about such things as meaning in life, relationships and perhaps even some kinds of transcendence, yet they do not identify any of this as 'spiritual' and I cannot impose this label on them. Much though I'd like to see this paradigm shift, if it ever occurs, I don't think it will be in my lifetime. Having said this, I think that it is also possible to argue that, in many ways, it has already taken place, even if only in a limited way.

Transcultural psychiatry, for example, has had a vision of the 'common humanity' at the heart of professional practice, albeit the place of spirituality and religion within this is variously construed and not entirely free from its own forms of reductionism (Antic, 2021). The diagnostic category 'Religious or Spiritual Problem', introduced into DSM since its fourth revision (Baccetto, 2023), does now give a significant space within which the spiritual dimensions of distress may be discussed in psychiatry without necessarily diagnosing pathology. Spirituality and religion find their way into most conceptualisations of the recovery approach and, most importantly of all in my view, patient-centred (or person-centred) care is now firmly established as foundational to the good professional practice of clinical psychiatry. Putting the patient at the centre of psychiatry, rather than the science, is arguably the best way of all to ensure that spirituality takes its rightful place at the heart of psychiatry. However, we cannot leave matters there because this still does not ensure that spirituality is given proper attention in practice, at least not in the secular Western world.

A Secular Age

Charles Taylor (2007) has drawn attention to how secularity has a way of viewing things (an 'imaginary' in his terminology) which is closed to transcendence. Secular societies adopt an immanent frame of reference. This 'immanent frame' includes, notably, an understanding of the 'buffered self', living in a social environment in which instrumental rationality is prized, and in which time is 'pervasively secular' (Taylor, 2007, p.542). To take just the first of these features of the immanent frame, the buffered, or bounded, self contrasts with the porous self of premodern society. As discussed earlier, this buffered self can more easily disengage from the surrounding world and is understood as less vulnerable to the influence of spiritual forces, whether good or evil. The buffered self faces a very different existential plight than does the porous self. It can step back from, and reflect on, the world around. Meaning and purpose are to be found within. The cost of this is the loss of an intimate connection with the world around us and with a transcendent order (something that Taylor goes on to discuss as a 'malaise of immanence').

The buffered self, according to Taylor, occupies a constructed social environment within which 'closed world structures' (CWSs) make transcendence a problematic topic. Taylor defines CWSs as 'ways of restricting our grasp of things which are not recognised as such' (Taylor, 2007, p.551). In particular, they are closed to transcendence and, further, they make this constructed way of looking at things seem natural, as though it is just how things are (rather than being a constructed worldview). Science, based on a materialist view of the world, is taken to be capable of explaining things, whilst religion is understood as mythology (in a bad sense of the word, not as meaningful and true): 'So religion emanates from a childish lack of courage. We need to stand up like men and face reality' (Taylor, 2007, p.561). The unbeliever, in contrast, is taken to be mature and courageous, and to have a (humanistic) grasp of reality as it 'really' is.

Taylor's understanding of secularity will be discussed further in Chapter 8 but, for now, the important thing to observe is that – if Taylor is correct – we cannot assume that patient-centred care will give adequate attention to spirituality in clinical practice in a secular health service. Patients are likely to find spirituality and religion difficult to talk about, perhaps even more so than other sensitive topics such as sex or death, and clinicians are likely to focus on the immanent concerns which were the preoccupation of their professional training. The boundary between the secular and the spiritual/religious, a fundamental feature of a health service in a secular society, makes spirituality a problematic topic for conversation. Even in the theoretically 'safe' space of the clinical consultation, patients can be afraid of censure because of the CWSs that – they fear – make transcendent topics off limits and subject to censure.

The perceived conflict between science and religion, to which Taylor alludes, will be further discussed in Chapter 4, but the way in which spirituality is excluded from clinical practice in psychiatry when, as I am arguing, it should be seen as central to it owes much to the unhelpful ways in which much of the popular debate has been conducted. Viewing theology or religion as incompatible with science in some way, rather than as complementary or in dialogue, easily leads to a perception that they cannot be discussed with scientists (including, here, clinicians as 'applied scientists') without fear of contradiction or dismissal. A more critical analysis of the relationship between science and theology in psychiatry is therefore needed and will be explored further in Chapter 4.

Faith Communities

This book looks at the entanglement of spirituality and psychiatry from the perspective of psychiatry. There are other perspectives, notably the perspectives of faith communities who struggle with the equal and opposite problem presented by the tangle. How may psychiatry, and mental health, be understood through the eye of faith? This is a real problem for some, given that psychiatry and spirituality/faith share many common concerns in relation to the human condition and the relief of suffering and distress. However, they share these concerns from very different standpoints, the one built largely upon a medical scientific foundation, with a focussed programme of the relief of sickness and suffering, and the other built upon a theological and philosophical foundation, with a broader quest for meaning, redemption and human flourishing. There is therefore plenty of scope for misunderstanding and suspicion.

There is a wide range of answers to this question of how psychiatry may be viewed from the perspective of religious faith, not only because there are many different religions but also because, within each faith tradition, there are a variety of different possible ways of engaging with the problem. Some adopt a very oppositional stance, emphasising boundaries between their faith community and a wider, spiritually dangerous world. Some adopt a much more integrative position. The former are much less likely to engage with secular health services and there may be significant reluctance to seek help from mental health professionals. For the latter there may be much less of a problem with engagement and access, but much more of a problem with questions around the impact of illness on faith and how to understand faith in relation to illness. This was very much the situation in which Jenny found herself in the story with which this chapter opened.

In order to try to improve mutual understanding, and remove unnecessary barriers, the American Psychiatric Association (in partnership with a number of other convening organisations) has established the Mental Health and Faith Community Partnership, to foster collaboration between psychiatrists and clergy (American Psychiatric Association, n. d.). This partnership promotes mutual education – of clergy about psychiatry, and of psychiatrists about spirituality and faith. In the current absence of anything similar in the UK and elsewhere, local collaborations between NHS mental health services and faith communities are all the more important.

Psychiatry

This is a book about psychiatry, but what exactly is psychiatry? At one level, the answer is quite simple. Psychiatry is a speciality within the wider field of medicine. Psychiatrists train to be doctors first and then specialise in what sometimes used to be called psychological medicine. However, psychological medicine – psychiatry – is not quite like other medical specialties. Take, for example, Nancy Andreasen's definition: 'Psychiatry is the medical specialty that studies and treats a variety of disorders that affect the mind—mental illnesses. Because our minds create our humanity and our sense of self, our specialty cares for illnesses that affect the core of our existence' (Andreasen, 1997, p.592).

This 'core of our existence' is what used to be called the soul. Etymologically, from the Greek, the word 'psychiatry' refers to a physician, or healer (*iatros*), of the soul, or mind (*psyche*). Ordained ministry in many parts of the Christian Church is also referred to as a 'cure of souls' and so, on an etymological basis, vocations to priesthood and psychiatry might be understood as much the same thing. In fact, we all know that in practice they are not, and problems occur when doctors, priests or patients begin to confuse the two. Andrew Sims, past president of the RCPsych and a strong advocate of the importance of addressing spirituality in psychiatry, suggested that, even though someone may tell much the same story, their reasons for telling it to a psychiatrist rather than a priest (or vice versa) are very different: 'The account is told to the psychiatrist with the hope that relief of psychic pain and distress will follow; it is told to the priest because the individual wants to make use of the priest's moral position and stance in relationship with God' (Sims, 1988, p.161). In Sims' understanding, the 'basis for a psychiatrist's knowledge of his patient is phenomenological; that is he uses his [or her] capacity for empathy as a delicate instrument to reveal the patient's own subjective experience' (Sims, 1988, p.161).

This empathic, phenomenological starting point for the work of the psychiatrist is just the beginning. Psychiatry draws upon a wide range of other disciplines, including, notably, the neurosciences, in order to understand the causes of a patient's distress. For some, it is this scientific basis for psychiatry that is fundamental, such that Samuel Guze, in a lecture at the Institute of Psychiatry in 1988, was able to assert that 'there is no such thing as a psychiatry that is too biological' (Guze, 1989, p.315). To be fair, by the end of the lecture he deftly weaves in an acknowledgement of the importance of psychotherapy, which he sees as in no way contradictory to his fundamental, biological premise. However, many would disagree completely with the biological emphasis and would argue that psychiatry has become much too biological over recent decades. For example, it has been suggested that 'Defining psychiatry as applied neuroscience valorizes the brain but urges on us a discipline that is both mindless and uncultured' (Kirmayer and Gold, 2011, p.308).

Others, finding the current 'technological paradigm' of psychiatry wanting, have argued that 'we need a radical shift in our understanding of what is at the heart (and perhaps soul) of mental health practice' (Bracken et al., 2012, p.432). Despite the language, they do not appear to be looking for a paradigm shift, of the kind discussed earlier, so much as a broadening of existing horizons: 'We are not seeking to replace one paradigm with another. A post-technological psychiatry will not abandon the tools of empirical science or reject medical and psychotherapeutic techniques but will start to position the ethical and hermeneutic aspects of our work as primary, thereby highlighting the importance of examining values, relationships, politics and the ethical basis of care and caring' (p.432). Kirmayer and Crafa (2014, p.1), similarly concerned about the over-emphasis on neuroscience, argue that what is needed is 'A multilevel, ecosocial approach to biobehavioral systems.' In such an approach, they argue, 'the coherence of the paradigm can come from its personal and social meaning rather than its reducibility to a discrete neural circuit'. Again, this is not a paradigm shift, more a combining of paradigms.

Concerns about reductionism and an over-emphasis on neuroscience are, as these examples show, now leading to a much broader vision of the grounds upon which psychiatry is built. This includes recognition of the importance of the humanities. For example, in an editorial in *Acta Psychiatrica Scandinavica*, some two decades ago, Tom Bolwig wrote: 'The humanities and arts are appropriate areas of study in interdisciplinary medicine, because within each patient, the physical, the psychological, emotional and spiritual are all inextricably linked' (Bolwig, 2006, p.381). Psychiatry is an art as well as a science (Chur-Hansen and Parker, 2005), and it concerns people understood in the full context of the human situation: 'At root, the neurobiological project in psychiatry finds its limit in the simple and often repeated fact: mental disorders are problems of persons, not of brains. Mental disorders are not problems of brains in labs, but of human beings in time, space, culture, and history' (Rose and Abi-Rached, 2013, p.140).

This broader view of things, which is essentially the basis for patient-centred care in psychiatry, is now gaining much more traction. However, spirituality and religion, as important aspects of 'culture and history' and the humanities more widely, not to mention the 'sense of self' of the vast majority of people worldwide, still repeatedly get forgotten. Even in Tom Bolwig's excellent editorial, from which I quoted just now, religion and theology are not mentioned at all, and spirituality is only mentioned in the passage that I quoted. Stephen Pattison has suggested that religion and theology are amongst the 'absent friends' of the medical humanities (Pattison, 2007). This is gradually changing, with critical exploration of the part that these absent friends play in the medical and health humanities (Slominski et al., 2026) and in psychiatry (Cook and Powell, 2022) increasingly acknowledged, but still as uncertain friends, rather than as loved members of the family. This book is therefore as much about the lost soul of psychiatry as it is about the souls of patients.

Tangles

Psychopathology is entangled with spiritual experience. Spirituality and religion are entangled with the very nature of psychiatry, and they are entangled with the biopsychosocial matrix of human life. Psychiatric training, at least in the RCPsych, but also in other national and international psychiatric associations, now promotes a person-centred holistic model of psychiatry and many patients (the vast majority worldwide) find spirituality and/or religion to be a core concern of life. The secular age in which we live, at least in the Western world, seeks to disentangle all of this, to relegate spirituality and religion to a private domain, to promote a pragmatic atheism in public life which makes it difficult or impossible to talk about spirituality and religion, and to build a barrier between the secular and the spiritual/religious domains of life. This same barrier intrudes upon the lives of people who belong to faith communities so as to make it more difficult for them to engage with mental health services. When they do engage, like Jenny, they face significant problems in trying to integrate their understanding of their faith and their illness in meaningful and health-promoting ways. Psychiatry, in its core concerns, has a vocation to help Jenny and others, not by disentangling, or even by a differential diagnosis between psychopathology and 'healthy' religious experience, but by recognising that a holistic and patient-centred model of practice is concerned with treatment of the psyche – mind and soul – in all its complex entanglements. The core concerns of psychiatry need to be much more closely aligned with the core concerns of patients, both immanent and transcendent. In order to do this, it needs to be more (not less) reflective on the core concerns of psychiatrists. Spirituality, entangled as it is with the biopsychosocial matrix within which psychiatry operates, offers a vision of something better, something more, which – although sometimes articulated only with difficulty – is at the heart of what patients are looking for when they enter treatment.

Chapter 2

The Spirituality of the Psychiatrist

If, as I have argued in Chapter 1, psychiatry and spirituality are entangled, how has this entanglement played out historically in the development of psychiatry as a clinical and academic discipline? How does it play out in the lives of psychiatrists and patients, in their interactions with one another in the clinic and on the ward? In seeking to find answers to these questions, I will explore the spirituality of the psychiatrist in this chapter, and a patient-centred approach to spirituality in Chapter 3. Perhaps in an ideal world I would have written these chapters the other way around, putting patients first. However, even in this age of co-production and patient advocacy, psychiatry has a world of thought which historically has been shaped by psychiatrists themselves, and it is necessary to understand that background in order to contextualise the spiritual challenges faced by patients today.

The spirituality of the psychiatrist is a much under-discussed subject, but it is important both because it may influence clinical practice, directly or indirectly, and because it may affect the well-being of the psychiatrist. For the purposes of this chapter, I am using the term 'spirituality' quite broadly, so I am interested here not just in what psychiatrists who self-identify as spiritual or religious may think but also in what those who do not may think. Antipathy and apathy towards spirituality are potentially just as important as acceptance and advocacy, whether for good or ill.

Research suggests that, as a generalisation, psychiatrists are less likely to be religious, and less likely to believe in God, than their patients (Cook, 2011a). This 'religiosity gap' does not necessarily imply that there is a 'spirituality gap' since we know that many people (at least in Western society) now identify as spiritual but not religious (SBNR) and there is reason to believe that a significant proportion of psychiatrists may adopt this self-identity (Peteet et al., 2016). At the time of writing, around a quarter of members of the Royal College of Psychiatrists are members of the Spirituality and Psychiatry Special Interest Group (SPSIG). Interest in spirituality, as evidenced by membership of such a group, does not necessarily imply that psychiatrists are either more or less spiritual than their patients. This said, there is every likelihood that psychiatrists understand spirituality and religion differently from their patients and it is important to better understand this 'epistemic gap' if we are to address some of the difficulties that psychiatrists and patients face in relation to psychiatry and spirituality.

How does psychiatry influence spirituality, and how does spirituality influence psychiatry, within the life and thought of the psychiatrist?[1] Asking these questions is not meant to

---

[1] I am asking the question here in respect to the psychiatrist as an individual person. Scientific debates will be considered in Chapter 4, and professional practice debates in relation to spirituality and psychiatry will be discussed in Chapter 8.

imply that self-identification as being spiritual or religious makes a doctor either a better or a worse psychiatrist. We know that the personal qualities of a doctor or therapist (such as interpersonal capacities) do impact outcomes (Heinonen and Nissen-Lie, 2020), and so it is possible that spiritual capacities – the skills needed to manage well the spiritual concerns of a patient – might also have an impact on outcomes, but spiritual capacities are not the same thing as self-identified spirituality/religiosity. It is quite possible that some atheist/agnostic psychiatrists might have as good (or better) personal qualities and skills in relation to managing the spiritual concerns of patients, at least insofar as the immediate clinical task is concerned. It all depends upon exactly what qualities/skills one might consider important, and exactly how one defines 'spiritual'. There is, however, evidence that 'more religious' psychiatrists are more likely to investigate the religious/spiritual concerns of their patients (Baetz et al., 2004; Menegatti-Chequini et al., 2020) and also (as will be discussed in Chapter 3) that some atheist/agnostic psychiatrists may handle the spiritual concerns of their patients badly.

It is also important to clarify that there is no implication here that guidance of regulatory bodies concerning good medical/psychiatric practice should be ignored. The General Medical Council (GMC), for example, in its guidance to doctors in *Personal Beliefs and Medical Practice*, states: 'You may talk about your own personal beliefs only if a patient asks you directly about them, or indicates they would welcome such a discussion. You must not impose your beliefs and values on patients, or cause distress by the inappropriate or insensitive expression of them' (General Medical Council, 2013, para. 31). This chapter is not concerned with boundary questions of this kind (which will be discussed in Chapter 8). The GMC guidance alludes to some of the possible dangers of talking about beliefs in such a way as to proselytise or otherwise cause distress. There is evidence that such abuses can and do occur and may adversely influence clinical decision-making (Galanter et al., 1991), and it is obviously good and proper for regulatory authorities to issue guidance designed to prevent this. However, the possibility that such conversations might sometimes be positively helpful is less often discussed, and failure to discuss such things with patients might also impact outcomes, for good or ill.

It is possible that training in, and clinical practice of, psychiatry influences the spirituality of the psychiatrist, and this might be either helpful or detrimental to the well-being of the psychiatrist. This is potentially important for health service delivery at a time when staff in mental health services are under enormous pressures at work as a result of staffing shortages, increased demand and stretched budgets. The spirituality of the psychiatrist may be an important coping resource at such times and may have a positive (or negative) effect upon working relationships with both colleagues and patients.

The spirituality of the psychiatrist may be an important factor, at least for some, in terms of a sense of vocational calling. Whilst relatively little systematic research seems to have been conducted on this, there is evidence that Christians and other religious people train to become doctors because of a religiously motivated desire to care for others in need (Carson and Koenig, 2004, pp.10–19; Yoon et al., 2015). On the other hand, psychiatry was for a century or more somewhat hostile to religion and this may have discouraged some doctors from pursuing a career in a supposedly 'godless' speciality.

Finally, the spirituality of the psychiatrist may also influence the way in which he or she understands and practises psychiatry, not just negatively as in cases of bad practice, but also positively, for example in terms of the impact that it has upon the therapeutic alliance with patients. Some patients appear to believe that this is very important, asking – for example – if they can see a Christian psychiatrist (Enoch, 2006), or else failing to engage with mental health services at all for fear that the psychiatrist (who, they expect, will not believe in God or be 'spiritual') will simply not understand their spiritual/religious concerns. A virtues-based approach has the potential to show the benefits of clinicians' religious and spiritual commitments to clinical practice, and highlights opportunities for us all to learn from one another how we may be better psychiatrists (Peteet, 2013).

Psychiatry and Spiritual Formation: A Personal View

My training in psychiatry was punctuated by some major life events. My first wife, Ruth, also a doctor, became ill whilst pregnant with our second child. After 18 months or so of intensive chemotherapy, radiotherapy and a bone marrow transplant, she eventually succumbed to her illness and died. My first publication in a medical journal, published less than a year after her death, was a personal reflection on this experience (Cook, 1985). Amongst other things, I was struck at the time by the one-way traffic of stories exchanged between doctor and patient. I knew about my patients' suffering and struggles, but they did not know about mine. Only many years later did I realise that although I did not tell my patients about my story, my story affected the way in which I related to the stories that they told me (Cook, 2020a). My story was different from theirs in many ways, and each human story is unique, but experiences of loss, suffering and spiritual struggles are also in certain ways universal. Over the years I hardly ever related my story to a patient, but I was aware that my suffering and that of my patients made a non-verbal connection of some kind; I would call it a spiritual connection.

My story was one of being brought up in a Christian family and, as I moved through teenage years to adulthood, gradually making Christian faith my own. A desire to help others, formed through Christian spirituality, was significant in my choice of vocation to become a doctor. My decision to become a psychiatrist was, in part, also an outworking of my Christian spirituality, although, in the 1980s, some other Christians were still somewhat perplexed as to why I – a Christian – would want to enter such a notoriously atheistic branch of medicine. I nearly changed my mind, thinking that other branches of medicine were more practical, with better and more tangible outcomes, but Ruth's illness diverted my attention away from possible career changes. Emerging from the other side of these experiences, after Ruth's death, brought new challenges, emotional, practical and spiritual.

On the one hand, Ruth's death evoked unsettling questions about whether or not the God to whom I had prayed daily for the preceding two years had really heard my prayers at all. How could I believe in a God who had not answered my prayers? On the other hand, my theological questions became entangled with my reading of Freud and my wider psychiatric training. It was easy to persuade myself that any faith I had once had must simply have been a form of wish fulfilment and that there was no God, other than as a projection of my innermost desires. My escape from this entanglement came when I read a quote from the Danish theologian Søren Kierkegaard (1813–1855) to the effect that anyone who does believe in God does so, at least in part, because they choose to believe.[2] I decided that I wanted to believe – and it was okay to want to believe. I had rational reasons for choosing belief, and the fact that I consciously wanted to believe, *pace* Freud, did not invalidate my beliefs.

---

[2] I have since tried to trace this quote without success. One Kierkegaard scholar told me that it sounded very like Kierkegaard, but he did not know where it might have come from.

At the time, this entanglement was troubling and unsettling. Reflecting back, I see it as the beginning of a process of exploration of the relationship between my theological and psychiatric understandings of the human condition. Had Ruth not died, this exploration may or may not still have taken place but, if it had, it would probably have followed a quite different path. Entangled as it was with my grief, it was a profoundly unsettling lesson in the importance of finding meaning and purpose amidst the most painful experience of my life at that time. From then on, the unconscious was both a place of encounter with the reality of God and a place in which it was necessary to be suspicious of the human capacity (and thus my capacity) to settle for illusions of God. (Perhaps for atheist colleagues there is a similar need to be suspicious of unconscious motivations for wanting and choosing not to believe?) As a psychotherapist friend would later tell me, images of God are born within the psyche but they are always less than God. If we are to grow spiritually, they must therefore die and be reborn, with each successive iteration of the cycle of birth, death and resurrection bringing us closer to the infinite, transcendent reality but never – in this world – actually reaching it. As Rowan Williams has reflected, both atheism and religious faith are as much about what we do *not* believe as they are about what we do believe (Williams, 2012, pp.281–291).

Three Historical Perspectives

Historically, much care of the mentally ill was provided within a religious context, but the birth of psychiatry as a medical speciality in the wake of the European Enlightenment emphasised its scientific credentials. Notwithstanding the religious motivation of some (e.g., the Tuke family, who established the Retreat at York), others saw psychiatry as standing over and against a religious worldview. Johann Christian Reil (1759–1813), who first coined the term 'psychiatry', disliked theology and wanted to emphasise the scientific nature of the discipline. There were thus, from the beginning, psychiatrists who more or less vigorously rejected religion in favour of science. Adoption of such a position was not necessarily to be unsympathetic to the religious views of one's patients, but neither was it a neutral stance. Other psychiatrists had positive views about religion, both personally and in relation to the mental well-being of their patients. Every psychiatrist has their own stance, and even if some have professed indifference, or have neglected the topic entirely, this in itself is a view on the matter. There is no view from nowhere.

Whilst there have been many and diverse historical perspectives, I have selected here three that I think have been historically influential, each represented by a particular clinician: Henry Maudsley, Sigmund Freud and Carl Jung. Respectively, these figures might be seen as adopting a pragmatic kind of atheism, an understanding of religion as pathology and a view of religion as beneficial to mental flourishing.

Henry Maudsley

An editor of the *Journal of Mental Science* and generous benefactor of the hospital that famously bears his name, Henry Maudsley (1835–1918) was a psychiatrist with strongly biological views on the causation of mental illness, and amongst the first to recognise an inherited component to mental disorders (Pantelidou and Demetriades, 2014). He became Superintendent of the Manchester Lunatic Asylum in 1858, at the age of only 23, but seems to have focussed on private practice as a means to accumulate wealth and to have been more influential by way of his philosophical and academic pursuits than as a clinician (Turner, 1988). Influenced by the scientific naturalism of his time, Maudsley took the view that religion was a creation of the human mind, owing to errors of reasoning, a view that we might now understand as falling within the cognitive science of religion (De Villaine, 2020). Events always have natural causes, according to Maudsley, and supposed supernatural causation only reflects the errors, limits and wrong assumptions of human understanding. Religious beliefs are a product of human imagination, which he contrasted with the sound reason and rationality of science. Supposed religious experiences he attributed to perceptual disorders, owing to brain dysfunction (e.g., epilepsy).

According to Aubrey Lewis, the publication in 1867 of Maudsley's first, most influential and most well-known book, *Physiology and Pathology of Mind*, 'marked a turning point in English psychiatry': 'it presaged the end of the period in which psychiatry rested on a magma of empirical observations and windy philosophizing, and it embodied a critical synthesis of biological and other scientific advances so far as they had an evident bearing on mental activity, in health and disease' (Lewis, 1951, p.269). Maudsley seems to have been a more complex figure than his theories on the origins of religion might suggest. According to George Savage, he was known to reject accusations of being opposed to religion and could see that it might be helpful to others, even if not to himself (Savage, 2018). This did not prevent him elsewhere from entertaining the possibility that religion might be the cause of mental disorder (Maudsley, [1895] 1979, pp.85–86). Lewis suggested that his views reflected the internal 'warring strains' attributable to 'the intellectual tough-minded inheritance from his father and the emotional, religious warmth from his mother' (Lewis, 1951, p.267). Whilst Maudsley was a positivist who rejected 'religion' at one level, he was not a hard materialist, more agnostic or deist than atheist, and was able to conclude that natural forces are all 'but modes of manifestation of one force – the Will of God – manifest in highest form and with least obscuration in the temple of man's body' (quoted by Lewis, 1951, p.264). It would therefore be unwise to oversimplify Maudsley's view of religion. However, it is nonetheless clear that Maudsley took a scientific view of psychiatry and, in this sense, he prefigured the stance that was to be adopted by much of the profession in the late twentieth and early twenty-first centuries.

Sigmund Freud

The figure most associated with an anti-religious stance within psychiatry was actually not a psychiatrist. Sigmund Freud (1856–1939), founder of psychoanalysis, was a neurologist, but his influence on thinking in relation to religion within psychiatry has been huge, arguably greater than that of any other individual figure. It is impossible here to do justice to the huge field of scholarship on Freud and religion, but equally it would be a grave omission not to say anything about him.[3]

Freud's parents, Jakob and Amalia, both came from Orthodox Jewish families, Jakob's being in the Haskalah tradition and Amalia's the Hasidic tradition. It is asserted that they had abandoned strict religious practices by the time their children were born (Jennings, 2024, p.13), but recent scholarship has questioned this view, at least in relation to Jakob

---

[3] A useful short account of Freud's views on religion may be found in Ross, 2022, pp.217–219. For a more detailed analysis, see Rizzuto, 1979, pp.13–39.

(Ross, 2022, p.97). Freud never practised Judaism, but his Jewish identity nevertheless seems to have been important to him and he would later describe himself as a 'godless Jew' (Meng and Freud, 1963, p.63). His arguments in support of this godlessness were, however, based on his psychological theories, rather than on scientific materialism or philosophy. God, he argued, was 'psychologically, nothing other than an exalted father . . . the roots of the need for religion are in the parental complex; the almighty and just God, and kindly Nature . . . or rather as revivals and restorations of the young child's ideas of them' (Freud, 1985b, p.216). The key elements of Freud's understanding of religion were thus related to child development (the Oedipus complex), the analogy that he saw between religion and neurosis, the psychological mechanism of projection and the contribution made by religion to civilisation (Banks, 1973, p.402).

In an essay on 'Obsessive Actions and Religious Practices', originally published in 1907, Freud ventured that he regarded obsessional neurosis 'as a pathological counterpart of the formation of a religion, and to describe that neurosis as an individual religiosity and religion as a universal obsessional neurosis' (Freud, 1985b, p.40). In 1910, in some paragraphs added to *The Psychopathology of Everyday Life* (published originally in 1901), Freud gives an account of unconscious motivation for forgetting, drawn from his own experience (Freud, 1975). The forgotten material was associated, in his mind, with a reversal of the biblical statement that 'God created man in His own image'; 'Man created God in his' (Freud, 1975, p.58). Later in *The Psychopathology of Everyday Life*, he refers to religion as a projection of unconscious material into the external world (Freud, 1975, p.321).

The Future of an Illusion, originally published in 1927, was probably Freud's most influential work on religion, although he was not very happy with it himself, and it has been criticised as un-Freudian and based largely on a very dated positivistic critique of religion (Dufresne, in Freud, 2012, p.13). Here, he argues that religion represents an infantile attachment to a protective father figure. Religion is thus an illusion, a regressive wishful thinking which provides a way of coping with the dangers and anxieties of adult life in the real world. As an illusion, it is not necessarily false, although Freud obviously thought that it was, but it is clearly very conveniently what we would wish: 'We tell ourselves that it would be very nice if there were a God – creator of the world and kind Providence – if there were a moral world order and a life in the hereafter, but it is quite obvious that all of this is just as we would wish' (Freud, 2012, p.95). We might note, in passing, that Freud does not consider the many ways in which this is exactly *not* as we would wish, and that the problems of reconciling a loving God with a suffering world (the theological problem of theodicy) represent a grave spiritual struggle which is avoided precisely by *not* believing.

Freud's friends also had some interesting, and differing, perspectives. Oskar Pfister, a Swiss pastor and lay analyst, in *The Illusion of a Future*, provided his counter-arguments (Freud, 2012). In the opening pages of his next book on the topic, *Civilisation and Its Discontents* (originally published in 1930), Freud refers to his correspondence with his friend Romaine Rollande. As Freud writes, for Rollande the true source of 'religious sentiments' lay in a certain kind of 'oceanic feeling', a sense of something limitless, eternal and unbounded (Freud, 1985a, p.251). Freud confessed that this was something unknown to him personally but that he recognised might be experienced by others. The question, as Freud rightly suggests, is how this subjective experience should properly be interpreted (Freud, 1985a, pp.251–252), but Freud clearly was not open to answering this question other than in terms of his own (arguably equally wishful) theories of human development (Bingaman, 2003, pp.12–13). In *Civilisation and*

Its Discontents, he goes further than in *The Future of an Illusion* and refers to religion as a 'mass-delusion' (Freud, 1985a, p.269).

In *Moses and Monotheism*, one of Freud's last published works (Freud, 1985a, pp.237–386), he returns to the topic of the phylogeny of religion, first addressed in *Totem and Taboo* (1913) (Freud, 1985a, pp.43–224). He argues (on highly speculative and almost completely unsubstantiated grounds) that Moses was an Egyptian, not a Hebrew, and that the origins of religion lay in the guilt associated with murder of a historical, primeval father. These theories rely heavily on a discredited Lamarckian view of evolution, contrary to Darwinism, by way of which this guilt is somehow passed down through the generations (Storr, 2001, p.107). I'm also left wondering whether Freud's atheism was not his own intellectual 'murder' of God as father figure, projected into a speculative primeval past. However, this is the problem with projections; it is like being in a hall of mirrors, that is, always difficult to know who is projecting what on to whom.

It is interesting that Freud gave so much attention in his published works to an 'illusion' that he considered to be completely false. Ironically, it may be argued that the reasons for this lay in his own psychological defences (Lamothe, 2003). Whereas Maudsley's atheism expressed itself in scientific rationalism, and a benign – if slightly patronising – acknowledgement of the possibility that religion might be good for others (even if not for him), Freud's psychoanalytic theories were altogether more complex. Claiming to be scientific, they were in fact impossible to verify by the scientific method. Offering a theory of the pathological basis for religious belief, they actually looked very like a kind of religion (Webster, 2005, pp.179, 389). However, they primarily focussed on Judaism and Christianity, completely neglecting Eastern religious traditions. They probably owe a greater debt than Freud was willing to acknowledge to the thinking of the philosopher Ludwig Feuerbach (1804–1872), whom Freud had read in some depth and whose work prefigured much of Freud's attitude towards religion (Levitt and Turgeon, 2009). Like Maudsley, Freud had a complete confidence in the superiority of intellectual rationalism over religion, but, unlike Maudsley, he seemed almost unable to comprehend the possible benefits of the religious experience of others.

Carl Jung

A more positive approach to religion was taken by one of Freud's pupils. Carl Jung (1875–1961),[4] son of a pastor in the Swiss Reformed Church, was born into a highly religious family. His maternal grandfather, also a pastor, was a theologian, Hebrew scholar and spiritualist. Several members of the family were identified as clairvoyant, and many of Carl's uncles were also pastors. His paternal grandfather (also Karl Gustav) was a distinguished physician and Freemason. Carl was, however, largely disappointed with his father, Paul, insofar as religious matters were concerned. Whereas the young Carl was intellectually stimulated by theological conversation with his maternal uncle, his father seemed studiously to avoid thinking critically about his faith. Carl's attempts to talk with him about such matters were a dismal failure: 'I did sometimes attempt to talk seriously with my father, but encountered an impatience and anxious defensiveness which puzzled me. Not until several years later did I come to understand that my poor father did not dare to

---

[4] For more detailed biographical information, the reader is referred to the following sources, upon which the present account is largely based: Jaffé et al., 1963 and Stevens, 1999, 2001.

think, because he was consumed by inward doubts. He was taking refuge from himself and therefore insisted on blind faith' (Jaffé et al., 1963, p.92).

Jung's early thinking about religion was driven as much by his mental experiences as by mere intellectual curiosity. *Memories, Dreams, Reflections* records his early dream of an underground phallus, which he interpreted in religious as well as psychological terms (Jaffé et al., 1963, pp.26–27). He struggled with fear of committing an unforgivable sin in his thoughts, which he then came to see as a test from God. As he ceased struggling with this train of thought, it culminated in a mental image of God defecating on Basil Cathedral, an experience which paradoxically brought him great relief (Jaffé et al., 1963, pp.52–58). Indeed, his memories of his childhood are full of his struggles with theological concerns, struggles which he resolved as much experientially as through intellectual endeavour. For Jung, religious experience was crucial; religion was not about doctrines and creeds, it was about experience: 'We might say, then, that the term "religion" designates the attitude peculiar to a consciousness which has been changed by experience of the numinosum' (Jung, 1986, p.8). The term 'numinosum' is one that Jung drew from the work of Rudolf Otto (1980), and refers to 'primary religious experience' (Stevens, 1999, p.248). Direct experiences of this kind were understood by Jung as experiences of the God image, which in turn was synonymous in his thinking with the Self archetype. For Jung, this experience was fundamental: 'Religious experience is absolute; it cannot be disputed. You can only say that you have never had such an experience, whereupon your opponent will reply: "Sorry, I have." And there your discussion will come to an end' (Jung, 1986, pp.104–105). In a famous television interview, when asked whether he believed in God, Jung replied simply, 'I know' (Stevens, 1999, p.249).

In *Memories, Dreams, Reflections*, writing of his childhood, Jung explained: 'Suddenly I understood that God was, for me at least, one of the most certain and immediate of experiences. After all, I didn't invent that horrible image about the cathedral. On the contrary, it was forced on me and I was compelled, with the utmost cruelty, to think it, and afterwards that inexpressible feeling of grace came to me' (Jaffé et al., 1963, p.80). Jung's understanding of God, as experiential, was therefore also fundamentally psychological and, as such, concerned much more with the 'God image' in the human psyche than with traditional theological debates about the ontological nature of God. As his thinking progressed, Jung came to see the God image as indistinguishable from symbols of the self (Colman, 2006, p.153). The Self (to be distinguished from the 'self', in common usage, and not at all the same thing as the ego) was central to Jung's psychology, representing both the totality of the psyche and its centre. Understood as an archetype (Colman, 2006, p.157), it was the manifestation of God within the soul (Stevens, 2001, p.61). The process of individuation, or realisation of the Self, is central to Jung's psychology and involves integration of the unconscious aspects of self into consciousness. Individuation is not a selfish or egotistical affair, but rather the central aim of analysis, and a process which might lead eventually to the opening of a window on to eternity (Stevens, 1999, pp.253–254).

In his 1942 essay 'A Psychological Approach to the Dogma of the Trinity' (Jung, 1986, pp.107–200), Jung controversially proposed that the Christian doctrine of the Trinity (that God is three persons, Father, Son and Holy Spirit, in one 'substance') should be expanded, to become a quaternity, by incorporation of the fourth person of Lucifer (Main, 2006, p.306). Just as Jung felt that it was psychologically important to integrate the unconscious, shadow aspects of the Self in order to achieve wholeness, so it was similarly necessary to acknowledge the shadow, or evil, aspects of the God image.

In *Answer to Job* (originally published in 1958), Jung went further in expressing his struggle with God – his grappling with the difficulty of reconciling the existence of God with evil in the world (the problem of theodicy). (Jung, 1986, pp.355–470). He argues that God projects evil on to his creation, and that the missing 'fourth element' of the Trinity is concerned not only with evil but with the feminine and the body (Main, 2006, p.307):

> God is not only to be loved, but also to be feared. He fills us with evil as well as with good, otherwise he would not need to be feared; and because he wants to become man, the uniting of his antinomy must take place in man . . . .. Since [man] has been granted an almost godlike power, he can no longer remain blind and unconscious. He must know something of God's nature and of metaphysical processes if he is to understand himself and thereby achieve gnosis of the Divine. (Jung, 1986, p.461)

Unsurprisingly, Jung's psychology of religion has been hugely controversial (Main, 2006, pp.310–315). He focusses primarily on monotheism, and on Western traditions, and (notwithstanding his emphasis on incorporating the feminine aspect of the divine) is at times androcentric and patriarchal. He does not always seem to properly understand theological constructs, such as the Augustinian view of evil as privation of the good (*privatio boni*). As with Freud's theories, Jung's are not amenable to refutation by the scientific method and arguably constitute a new kind of religion in themselves. However, if they are a religion, they are one in which religion itself is reduced to psychology.

Three Types of Entanglement

The atheisms of Maudsley and Freud look very different, with the former more willing than the latter to see that religion could perhaps be helpful in the lives of some of his patients. Maudsley's scientific rationalism much more closely approximates to that tendency within psychiatry today to operate on the basis of a 'pragmatic atheism'. Roughly stated, we don't talk about God in psychiatric practice because – as the argument goes – we don't need to. We can understand all that we need to about how to help our patients without reference to God. Paradoxically, this is exactly not what Freud had in mind. In order to understand the neurosis of the religious patient, one has to recognise that God is an illusion, a form of wish fulfilment. Only once we have recognised this can we truly dispense with God. There are thus two possible kinds of atheist/agnostic entanglement of psychiatry with religion. One imposes a pragmatic atheism, on the basis of a scientific materialism which considers religion irrelevant. The other argues more vigorously that religion is a part of the problem, a pathology which needs to be addressed if not in treatment then certainly in academic discourse.

For Jung, God was a matter of human experience, a feature of the human psyche, and therefore necessary to discuss in clinical practice not in order to dispense with belief but in order to know oneself better. Whilst always arguing that he was not engaged in metaphysical speculations about the actual nature of God, he still managed to express highly original, controversial and complex views, which looked and sounded very much like theology. For Jung, religion was entangled with psychiatry not because it was a part of the pathology but because it was a part of the remedy.

Three More Recent Examples

Psychiatry has moved on since Jung died in 1961, but it continues to reflect a plurality of views concerning its scientific foundations, its engagements with mind and brain, and its entanglements with spirituality and religion. As Anthony Clare famously argued, psychiatry is 'in dissent'. Whilst I would argue that the three basic options for engaging with religion, as illustrated by Maudsley, Freud and Jung, are still alive and well, they are now manifested in countless different ways. I have chosen just three examples for further consideration here: Frank Lake, Mark Epstein and Olga Kharitidi. These choices have been made with a view to diversity and availability of relevant published sources in which psychiatrists' beliefs have been related to their psychiatric practice. However, many others might have been chosen, including some who have had some very interesting things to say about spirituality/religion in relation to psychiatry, such as Viktor Frankl (1905–1997), Elisabeth Kübler-Ross (1926–2004), Ana-Maria Rizzuto (b. 1932), Gerald May (1940–2005), Harold Koenig (b. 1951), Dhinesh Bhugra (b. 1952) and Wafa Sultan (b. 1958), to name but a few.

Frank Lake

Founder of the Clinical Theology Association (now the Bridge Pastoral Foundation), Frank Lake (1914–1982) trained originally in tropical medicine and was a missionary in India from 1939 to 1950.[5] Whilst working as superintendent of the Christian Medical College at Madras, he became interested in psychiatry and, returning to England, he retrained in psychiatry, gaining his diploma in psychological medicine in 1958. His major work, *Clinical Theology* (Lake, 1966), in which he 'correlates theological and psychiatric data' (p.xv), was published in 1966. He saw himself as an 'amateur theologian' (p.xv) and his approach was clearly evangelical. However, the 'central empirical finding' of his 'clinical theological studies' is deeply catholic (in the sense of being universally Christian) in its focus on the incarnation of Christ:

> It is this, that in the severest forms of mental pain, those which underlie the schizoid position, in which depth analysis shows that being-itself is lost, under conditions of trans-marginal stress, and the paranoid position, in which all well-being, rights, and sustenance have been similarly lost, there is a close correspondence between the agony of the human spirit as it endures these ultimate injuries, and the agony of Christ in his crucifixion. (pp.xvi–xvii)

Lake's approach to psychiatry was (as the quote demonstrates) psychoanalytic, influenced by Harry Guntrip, Melanie Klein, Donald Winnicott and Ronald Laing. Chapter headings in *Clinical Theology* almost entirely reflect psychoanalytic concerns, rather than theological themes, and a massive 371 pages, almost a third of the book, is given over to a study of schizoid personalities. *Clinical Theology* is certainly informed by psychoanalytic thinking. It is less clear that the interdisciplinary dialogue works well in the other direction.

Clinical Theology is prolix, and this makes it difficult to evaluate the engagement between psychiatry and theology that it offers. To take just a few examples, in a chapter on dissociative reactions it is said early on that 'The technical name for religious dissociation is hypocrisy' (Lake, 1966, p.461) and the next 10 pages explore biblical examples including Jesus's condemnation of the pharisees, saints Peter and Paul, as well as a broad category of Anglican clergy. In the chapter on phobic reactions, an early link is made between a *privatio*

---

[5] For a biography and helpful review of Lake's work, see Peters, 1989.

boni in infancy (identified as perinatal trauma) and the Augustinian doctrine of evil as *privatio boni*. At the beginning of the long chapter on schizoid personalities, 14 reasons are offered for the importance of this topic to clinical theology, including assertions that schizoid states often take on a religious 'flavour', purported links with the occult, a tendency of 'schizoid theologians' to rely too heavily on introspection, and the need for 'an entirely new dynamic system to effect behavioural change', which Lake finds in 'Death to the self by identification with the death of Christ' (p.556). The links made between psychoanalytic thought and theology are thus diverse, provocative and debatable.

Lake was also a keen advocate of LSD abreaction (using lysergic acid diethylamide – LSD-25) to facilitate regression to address perinatal trauma (Campbell, 2019, pp.166–167). Whilst he was theologically conservative, clinical theology, as an approach to pastoral care and counselling, was a radical innovation. *Clinical Theology* has been described by one leading pastoral theologian as a 'cult book', with Lake as charismatic leader of the cult (Campbell, 2019). Thousands of clergy and others attended his popular training seminars up and down the country and Lake influenced the pastoral formation of a whole generation of clergy. His emphasis on perinatal trauma is no longer considered orthodox within psychiatry (if, indeed, it ever was); his approach to psychiatry generally seems very dated now; and his method of bringing together science and theology was applauded by some, but seen as illogical by others (Lilley et al., 2016, p.24). The influence of clinical theology was undoubtedly far greater within the church than within psychiatry, where it was negligible, and it has waned considerably since Lake's death. However, the Bridge Pastoral Foundation continues to provide training based on a holistic approach to pastoral care.

Mark Epstein

A psychiatrist in private practice in New York, Mark Epstein (b. 1953) is the author of a series of books on Buddhism and psychoanalytic psychotherapy. Introduced to Buddhism even before commencing training at medical school, he evaluated his training as a psychiatrist through the 'prism' of Buddhism:

> I tended to look at everything I was learning about therapy through the prism or lens of Buddhist thought. Buddhism made therapy make sense to me. I came to see that Western psychotherapy has the potential to be a vehicle of awakening just as meditation can be. It is another way of uncovering and confronting the egocentric preoccupations that keep us from living a more fulfilling life. (Epstein, 2022, pp.43–44)

Despite this, he initially kept his Buddhist beliefs apart from his clinical work: 'But as he became more forthcoming with his patients about his personal spiritual leanings, he was surprised to find how many of them were eager to learn more. The divisions between the psychological, emotional, and the spiritual, he soon realized, were not as distinct as one might think' (Epstein, 2022, back cover).

Although Buddhism is undoubtedly one of the world's major religions, it is generally also atheistic, a religion without belief in any divinity. Epstein is thus plausibly able to self-identify as SBNR (Epstein, 2022, p.6). The thoroughly integrated understanding of Buddhism and psychoanalysis that emerges from Epstein's later writings provides both a psychoanalytic perspective on the life and teachings of the Buddha and a Buddhist perspective on psychoanalysis. For Epstein, Freud's understanding of the oceanic feeling 'reduced spiritual experience to a resurrection of infantile oneness with the mother at the breast' (Epstein, 2013, p.16). Epstein believes that:

> Freud, in looking solely through the eyes of a needy infant, was missing the boat. Buddhist mindfulness, like therapy, is built on the cultivation not just of an infant's consciousness but also of a mother's. It would be more accurate to say that it allows a return of the underlying rapport that binds us to each other as first expressed in mother-child union. (Epstein, 2022, p.280)

The four noble truths of Buddhism are concerned with suffering: the realistic view of suffering, its cause, its end and the noble eightfold path as the way out of suffering. For Epstein, both mindfulness, as a component of the eightfold path, and therapy have a part to play in helping us come to terms with suffering and with the nature of reality (p.280). Meditation and psychotherapy both 'encourage a willingness to face the horrors of life, those that dwell within and those imposed from without, with a courage and trust that can be hard to otherwise muster' (Epstein, 2022, p.288).

In *The Zen of Therapy* (2022), Epstein acknowledges that it is difficult to articulate exactly how Buddhism influences his work with his patients. One of his patients suggested that his method is one of '"friendly conversation" with occasional moments of illumination' (p.263) and Epstein, whilst acknowledging this as a good answer, yet seeks to identify something more, eventually settling on kindness and 'non-interfering attentiveness' (p.268). He goes on to talk about 'meditative sensibility' (p.268), 'learning by unlearning' (p.270) and a 'movement from grievance to gratitude' (p.272). What is clearly not in doubt is that Buddhism is deeply entangled with psychoanalysis in his practice of psychiatry.

Olga Kharitidi

Born in Siberia, Olga Kharitidi (b. 1960) worked for many years during the Soviet era in a mental hospital at Novosibirsk before later moving to the USA. In her autobiographical account of her journey into shamanism, *Entering the Circle* (Kharitidi, 1996), she describes her initial unexpected experiences in the Altai mountains and her subsequent spiritual quest, with its lasting impact on her clinical practice. Kharitidi had a variety of spiritual encounters that might be variously described as visions, lucid dreams or perhaps dissociative states. Her own account of her experience is one of changing identity, brought about by her 'Spirit Twin' who facilitates her vocation to heal and to become her true self. The religious context for Kharitidi's story might best be described as neo-shamanism, a strand of New Age spirituality which draws on ancient religious traditions of shamanism but which eschews the traditions and institutions of the major Western faith traditions, whilst at the same time claiming to be the fount of all great religions (Selberg, 2001, 2010, pp.231–232).

Some have questioned the 'anomalous elements' in Kharitidi's account (Hammer, 2004, pp.90–91), or have drawn unfavourable parallels with the discredited popular accounts of shamanism published by Carlos Castaneda (1925–1998) (Vinogradov, 2008, pp.41–42). However, there seems no reason to doubt the fundamental historical veracity of Kharitidi's autobiography and it is hard to see how one can question the content of highly subjective experiences (as opposed to the interpretation of these experiences, which of course may be highly questionable). In a second book, *Master of Lucid Dreams* (2001), Kharitidi makes a trip to Uzbekistan, where she is introduced to another strand of shamanism, associated with an ancient local religious tradition, in which she finds healing for her own trauma through a process of lucid dreaming. As with the first book, the message is very much in the narrative, and is not engaged with in a critical academic way. Frustratingly, she does not explore possible interpretations of her experiences in the light of Freud or Jung. Most psychiatrists will undoubtedly want to know more about the phenomenology of Kharitidi's experiences and will want empirical evidence to support the accounts of healing brought about by shamanic practices. However, they will also find no shortage of plausible psychological explanations for most of the healings that she describes, and she clearly writes for a popular lay audience, not a critical medical readership.

Three More Tangles

In very different ways, Lake, Epstein and Kharitidi each achieve a synthesis of their psychiatric and theological (or, for Epstein, atheological) ways of thinking about the human condition and the nature of their work as psychiatrists. The thinking of Lake and Epstein about psychiatry was from the outset formed by their prior religious beliefs. Neither of them fundamentally deviated from these prior beliefs, although they both introduced a large dose of psychoanalytic theory into, respectively, Christianity and Buddhism. For Kharitidi, there seems to have been a more intertwined evolution of her thinking in which (as for Jung, and for me) experience was important in shaping both her spirituality and her psychiatry. For all three, this process of epistemic synthesis seems to have been clinically creative and beneficent, although it has also stretched the boundaries – perhaps further than some might think is properly professional (a topic to which we shall return in Chapter 8).

Psychiatrists on Religion

Given these entanglements, how did anyone ever suppose that psychiatry can be understood from an entirely secular perspective, devoid of the views of the psychiatrist on theology or religion? Obviously much has to do with the European Enlightenment, the pervasive influence of figures such as Freud and Maudsley, and the 'closed world structures' (CWSs) of secularity which make things seem 'obvious' when they are not. Things may well seem very different in the non-Western world. A strong emphasis on the scientific credentials of psychiatry marginalises the concerns that theology and the medical humanities have with such things as meaning-making or a transcendent frame of reference. Unfortunately, this simultaneously marginalises the concerns of patients who struggle to make spiritual sense of their suffering and for whom spiritual/religious beliefs are inevitably entangled with psychopathology. It also tends to make mental health professionals, whose training often includes little or nothing about theology, religion or spirituality, blind to the ways in which their own understandings of mental illness may differ radically from those of their patients.

These entanglements are complex, and quite different for each of the psychiatrists considered in this chapter (my own experiences included). Maudsley was quite right to remind us of the importance of science and biology in psychiatry, and Freud drew attention to the very real ways in which religion may be unconsciously motivated. Jung, Lake, Epstein and Kharitidi have positive, but also widely varying accounts of religion to offer. How can psychiatry respond constructively to the almost infinitely variable entangling of spirituality and psychiatry amongst psychiatrists, in a way that is respectful of the spirituality of patients and contributory to their recovery? It is to this question that we must turn in Chapter 3.

Patient-Centred Spirituality

Spirituality plays a significant part in the lives of many people with mental health difficulties and yet, as users of mental health services, they do not always find that their spiritual concerns are taken seriously (Macmin and Foskett, 2004; Milner et al., 2020). Positive religious coping plays an important part in managing mental illness, and is associated with reduced symptoms, positive psychological adjustment and better outcomes (Tepper et al., 2001; Yangarber-Hicks, 2004; Rosmarin et al., 2013).[1] Autobiographical accounts of experiences of mental illness in the context of faith show that patients have great difficulty in making spiritual sense of their illness, and that illness also impacts upon the experience of faith and spirituality (e.g., Wield, 2012; Hastings, 2020). A person-centred approach to psychiatry should therefore take into account a patient's spirituality on its own terms, within the context of their faith or worldview, and consider how this may be utilised positively in treatment planning.

Two clinical cases will be used as a focus in this chapter in order to facilitate reflection upon what patient-centred spirituality might look like. In the first, spirituality was not explicitly mentioned at all but, it will be argued, was at the heart of the interaction between psychiatrist and patient. In the second, spirituality/religion explicitly influenced both the interactions with clinical staff and the presentation of the illness. Patient-centred spirituality creates a space within which clinician and patient can have existentially meaningful conversations about suffering and pain, whether or not the language used is explicitly spiritual/religious.

Sarah

As I related in Chapter 2, psychiatry had a significant impact on my spirituality during and after my training. My spirituality also had a profound impact upon my clinical practice, although it was many years before I fully appreciated this. Sometimes I worked with patients, or relatives of patients, who were bereaved, whose suffering took a similar shape to mine. In other cases, the suffering of my patients was far removed from my own experience. Either way, and even though I hardly ever said anything about my own story, I found an emotional resonance with those for whom I cared, and a sensitivity to the kinds of vocabulary on which I might draw in speaking to them. In itself, this might not necessarily be understood as spirituality, more psychology, but in practice it became very difficult to disentangle the two. Spiritual concerns cannot fully be expressed without recourse to psychological language, and some supposedly psychological conversations seem to have a very spiritual feel to them, even if the language of spirituality is not explicitly

---

[1] Negative religious coping will be discussed in Chapter 6.

employed. An example of the latter kind, where spirituality was not explicit, arose in my work as an addiction psychiatrist, only a year or two before I retired from clinical practice.

A young woman in her thirties, I will call her Sarah, attended our clinic to talk about her drinking problems. As was so often the case with patients in my clinic, Sarah's drinking was in large part a dysfunctional coping strategy. It blotted out painful memories and difficult feelings and enabled her not to confront her problems directly. For whatever reason (members of AA might call it her 'rock-bottom' experience) she had now accepted that she needed help and had taken first steps towards facing up to the deeply painful circumstances that lay behind her heavy drinking. Initially, she had spoken to one of the female nursing staff, who had then asked me to come and see her. Conversation amongst the three of us rapidly focussed not on the drinking behaviour but on the extensive abuse that this young woman had suffered at the hands of the men in her life. She told us about the physical and sexual abuse that she had experienced at the hands of her father, her brothers and multiple partners. As she told us the story, she became increasingly angry and eventually the passion in her voice and on her face overflowed. 'Sometimes, I just want to go out onto the street and stick a knife into every man that I meet.' She paused, looked at me and smiled. 'But not you.' I could have cried. I can't remember exactly what I had said up until that point in the conversation, and I think I had done a lot more listening than speaking, but somehow this woman who had suffered so much at the hands of the men around her had felt able to share with me – yet another man – her anger, her pain and, even more importantly, her shattered trust. Even now, years later, this exchange brings tears to my eyes. That morning, in the clinic, I was aware of the enormous privilege of being a psychiatrist, and grateful that I had at least provided a safe space within which one wounded woman could begin her journey to recovery. For me, this was a very spiritual moment, and one for which I am profoundly grateful.

I know other psychiatrists will agree that being a psychiatrist is a great privilege, but some may challenge the need to resort to the language of spirituality to describe my interaction with Sarah. I had listened well – just as I had been trained to do. I had provided a safe space in which she could tell her story. I had worked collaboratively with a nursing colleague who had already done a lot of important groundwork. God was not mentioned – nor was spirituality of any kind. So, why do I think that this was a spiritual encounter? I have wondered about this since, and struggled to articulate a coherent answer that works convincingly within the broader professional context. As a Christian, I have some theological answers, concerned with the teachings of Jesus that insofar as we do things for another human being in need – any human being – we do them for him.[2] In this way, my Christian theology and spirituality impact upon my experience and interpretation of that clinical encounter. My personal narrative and my theological narrative are entangled. Whether or not this was a spiritual encounter for Sarah, it was for me. So perhaps it was my Christian faith and my life experiences that shaped my understanding of my interaction with Sarah as having a spiritual quality, whereas it would not have been for anyone else concerned, Sarah included? But what about the psychiatric narrative? Can my encounter with Sarah be understood as spiritual in some broader way that makes sense within a secular world of mental health care?

---

[2] This derives from a parable told by Jesus in Matthew 25:31–46. I have previously argued that this passage has particular relevance for a Christian theology of mental health, in Cook, 2013b, pp. 217–218.

One possible answer to my question may be found within my subspeciality of addiction psychiatry, where the popularity of the 'spiritual but not religious' approach of Alcoholics Anonymous and its sister organisations, based upon the 12-step programme, has had huge impact. Although 12-step programmes are fundamentally about mutual help, and not professionally led, 12-step facilitation, which has a strong research evidence base, has operated within medically led services in such a way as to allow professional staff to recommend such programmes and support their patients as they pursue recovery within them. Religiously based programmes of recovery, also operating outside psychiatric services, have also produced good results. Although I did not refer Sarah to AA or a religiously based programme (and some might argue that I should have done, although this did not seem to me to be the right moment to do so), there is a greater acceptance of the need to talk about spiritual aspects of recovery in addictions services. Similar options do not exist for patients in general adult psychiatry, at least not in most Western clinical contexts, although a recent review of religion-based interventions for mental disorders, including anxiety, depression, psychological stress and addiction, suggested that such interventions are effective and worthy of further study (Kurhade et al., 2022).[3] So perhaps addiction psychiatry has something to offer psychiatry in general; perhaps spirituality/religion can and should make sense of clinical encounters within a wider world of mental health care?

Another possible answer to my question may be found in relation to an understanding of spirituality as concerned with how people deal with suffering. There are many definitions of spirituality but, in practice, spirituality often finds expression in relation to emotionally painful human experiences: loss, physical or mental illness, recovery from addiction, death and trauma. Such experiences may also be the opportunity for loss of faith but, for those who retain faith, post-traumatic growth (Shaw et al., 2005) and a search for meaning often draws upon spiritual or religious frameworks of understanding. I say this partly in relation to my own experience, but also in relation to countless patients with whom I worked over the years who found the spirituality of 12-step programmes helpful. Similarly, within the wider domain of mental health care, many patients identify the spiritual aspects of their recovery as being important to them. Spirituality and religiosity offer valuable resources for coping in the face of adversity. On this basis, patient-centred spirituality can and should make sense within the wider world of healthcare simply because it is the patient perspective that is at the centre. In this case, Sarah alone would be the arbiter of whether or not our conversation in the clinic that day was spiritually significant.

The Psychiatrist's Perspective

Perhaps psychiatrists who, like me, identify as spiritual (whether or not religious) may be more likely to recognise the value of spirituality/religion as coping resources than those who are neither spiritual nor religious? Certainly, the psychiatrist influenced by the traditional Freudian view of religion as a form of neurosis would not be likely to promote spiritual/religious coping. Nor does a deterministic and reductionistic view of human nature help. For example, I have heard it said by one psychiatrist that it is difficult with integrity to encourage patients to engage with 12-step programmes, notwithstanding evidence that they might actually be helpful to them, if you do not yourself 'believe' in them. In such situations,

---

[3] The review focussed on Islam, Hinduism, Christianity, Buddhism and Sikhism, but found no relevant studies of interventions based on Hinduism.

ironically, the spiritual/theological non-beliefs of the professional seem to override faith in the empirical research evidence base of medicine. So, I am left wondering, do I simply 'import' spirituality into my understanding of the clinical consultation because it is important to me? If so, do I do things any differently – for better or worse – because I do so?

I am struck by Mark Epstein's reflections on his clinical work (discussed in Chapter 2), where he seems to be asking similar questions of himself as a Buddhist.

> I know that Buddhism has been and remains a major influence in my work. Having evolved my own style as a therapist, I have come to trust myself to find my way with the people who come to see me. For this book, I set myself the task of probing my own process more deeply. Can I explain what Buddhism is bringing to the table? I have always wanted it to come through wordlessly. Is it? Or are my words important too? (Epstein, 2022, p.56)

In the clinical cases that he reports, much of Epstein's Buddhism is indeed 'wordlessly' conveyed – rather as my theology of encountering Christ in my patients was never verbalised in my interactions with them. However, sometimes he is quite explicit. Take, for example, his description of his working with Jack, where he talks about the Buddhist bodhisattva of compassion Kuan Yin (Epstein, 2022, p.65), his recommendation to Violette of a Buddhist book on tantric sex (pp.92–95), or his conversation with David about the Buddhist demi-god Mara (pp.142–147). In one consultation he actually talks to his patient about Jesus (pp.135–137, 165) and in another about the *I Ching* of Taoism (pp.257–262). If a Buddhist can talk to his patients about Jesus, then is it permissible also for a Christian to do so? Of course, Epstein is in private practice in the USA, and things are different within a publicly funded health service such as the National Health Service in the UK, but it is nonetheless important to reflect, across international borders, on the important ways in which spirituality/religion might be beneficially integrated into clinical practice. Are we missing something important if we exclude such topics from clinical interactions? Before returning to this question, another question arises. Is there a spirituality within psychiatry that, rather like my conversation with Sarah, expresses itself implicitly and without recourse to external traditions such as Buddhism or Christianity?

The Spirituality within Psychiatry

The problem with spirituality as a dependent variable, when it comes to quantitative research, is that it is confounded with independent psychological variables such as meaning, hope, peace, harmony and subjective well-being (Koenig, 2008a). This is not a problem for clinical work, or for qualitative research, where spirituality can be expressed in diverse ways, according to the understanding of the patient or research subject concerned. However, it does raise the question of whether or not the meaning of the term can be completely captured within a psychological vocabulary, or whether in fact there is something about it that cannot be expressed in such terms. If it is completely reducible to a psychological vocabulary, then perhaps (although not necessarily) the term is redundant as far as psychiatry is concerned?

The most helpful agnostic-atheist argument in support of the importance of spirituality that I have come across in relation to mental health has been the view comprehensively laid out by Jeremy Holmes (2024). In his exploration of the complex and contested definitions of spirituality, Holmes suggests that 'the term affirms that there are dimensions to life which resist representation or description, yet which shape what really matters to us' (p.27) and that 'the term captures the *emergent patterns of meaning and connectedness* which shape our beliefs, behaviour, and relationships' (p.27, original emphasis preserved). He goes on to develop an understanding of spirituality and psychotherapy as offering 'transitional space' within which to address some of the key psycho-spiritual tasks that human beings face. Holmes argues his case by recourse to Karl Friston's model of free energy minimisation (FEM), although I'm not sure that this is a necessary theoretical premise. Whether or not one subscribes to theories of FEM, it is possible to understand the human condition as negotiating a tension between, on the one hand, the chaos, uncertainties, threats and dangers of a world that is largely outside our control and, on the other hand, narratives that provide meaning and make the world more predictable and subject to our own agency and control.

Both psychotherapy and spirituality offer a transitional space within which it is possible to explore our fears and fantasies safely in such a way as to reduce anxiety and find meaning. Transitional space, a concept introduced by Donald Winnicott, encompasses the tensions between, on the one hand, an internal world of memories, fantasies, hopes and expectations and, on the other hand, the realities of our internal and external environments. In transitional space we can explore our dreams, be creative and imagine new possibilities (Holmes, 2024, p.20). Understood according to this view, Sarah's willingness to express to me and my nursing colleague the fantasy that she wanted to 'stick a knife into every man that she met' was both a spiritual and a psychological way of expressing her pain and a request to us, as health professionals, to help her in managing her painful inner world. It was also a request to assist her in her search for a way to make her external world safer, or at least less dangerous, and more meaningful.

Holmes goes on to say that 'Spirituality rather arises out of states of mind – cognitive and affective – that bring together top-down values with bottom-up impulses, and so helps people live with and to an extent transcend pervasive uncertainty' (Holmes, 2024, p.98). He suggests that the concept of mentalising offers something similar within psychotherapy. Mentalising refers to 'a subject's capacity to "see oneself from the outside and others from the inside"' (p.102). Spirituality is fundamentally concerned with adopting a 'viewpoint outside the self' (p.105). This viewpoint need not be conceived of in theistic terms. For members of Alcoholics Anonymous, the important consideration was (and is) that their Higher Power is simply not the self, and that it is decentring of the self, affirming that I am 'not God', that really matters (Kurtz, 1991). Nor is a belief in God always associated with a mentalising perspective. Holmes, drawing on Rowan Williams (2012, pp.15–16), cautions that fundamentalist religion, in eliminating uncertainty, undermines the very nature of spirituality. Spirituality is concerned with negative capability, humility and awareness of limitations and of the constraints of one's own perspective.

Whereas Holmes sees mentalising as offering transitional space, with a similar indebtedness to Winnicott, Epstein sees meditation as a transitional object (Epstein, 2022, pp.236–237). A transitional object is, as Epstein writes, 'both "me" and "not-me"' (p.236). Mentalising and meditation are not exactly the same thing, but they are very closely related. Epstein's understanding of meditation, as a Buddhist, does not have a theological reference. However, for those of us that are theists, I think that the ambiguity is helpful. I am 'not God', as members of AA would remind us, but this statement has to be nuanced by theological assertions (at least in Christianity, but also in other religions) that God is omnipresent. God is found deeply within, and not just in the external world or in some remotely removed transcendent place. Meditation, mindfulness and prayer blur boundaries and create a liminal space within which we may encounter the divine.

Gerald May (1982, pp.22–24), an American psychiatrist and Christian, who later in life worked as a spiritual director and retreat director, suggests that there are many kinds of spirituality, but two extreme representations: an affective way of talking about spirituality, which emphasises experience, and a metaphysical way, which emphasises interpretation. The approaches taken by Holmes and Epstein have elements of both but tend to focus on the experience and on psychoanalytic interpretation. Others (e.g., Lake or Kharitidi – see the discussion in Chapter 2) might offer a more theological interpretation of both their own and their patients' experiences, but whereas the account of the experience has to be taken at face value (unless there is any reason to suspect dissimulation), there is freedom to interpret experiences differently.

I realise that neither I nor Jeremy Holmes will persuade every psychiatrist or psychotherapist that the word 'spirituality' is a helpful or necessary one, but perhaps that does not matter so much as the willingness to use it in conversation with patients who do find it helpful. If 'a rose is a rose by any other name', then perhaps also conversations about suffering, meaning and existential concerns are still helpful in every way that matters (psychologically and spiritually), even if they are not explicitly referred to as 'spiritual'. Even if conversation about spirituality can be completely reduced to psychological terms, psychology cannot similarly be reduced entirely to spirituality. What does matter is that psychologists and psychotherapists should be able to talk about things like meaning and purpose in life, hope, peace and gratitude, and that it is important that they should not forget to do so. In clinical practice, these conversations will usually be had in the language preferred by the patient, which may be the language of spirituality, or of a particular religious tradition, or perhaps in some other language altogether. Retention of the term spirituality is important, but mainly because it helps us not to forget to have these conversations when patients want to have them. Generally (but certainly not always) I suspect that psychiatrists who self-identify as spiritual are less likely to forget the need for these conversations.

Hannah

I was asked to see Hannah by a colleague. She had a long history of bipolar disorder, with one episode of mania managed on an inpatient basis some years earlier. For some years now she had suffered chronic depressive symptoms which had not responded to medication. She said she wanted to speak to a 'Christian psychiatrist' and didn't want to talk about her faith to either the nurses or the doctors who were treating her, as she was convinced that they would simply see this as part of her illness. She was also not happy talking to the mental health chaplain. She had read something that he had written which she did not agree with, and I got the impression that she considered him in some way unorthodox, perhaps 'heretical', or otherwise beyond the pale.

When I met with Hannah and her partner she came across as quiet and somewhat withdrawn but was still able to tell me about her faith, her illness, her marriage and her church. Her Christian faith was, or at least had been, the motivating force in her life. She had no specifically spiritual/religious problems, except insofar as everything was coloured by her depressive outlook on life. God and church were no exception to this. She said that her 'mind was empty' and this emptiness seemed to have affected her relationship with God who was not so much angry with her or against her as uninterested and distant. She wondered whether she might be a victim of witchcraft. This belief was not held with delusional intensity and was congruent with beliefs held within the charismatic evangelical church to which she belonged where much of life was interpreted through a theological worldview of the influence of supernatural spiritual forces (both good and bad) upon human life and well-being. She had stopped attending church, partly because she lacked motivation but also because she felt that she could not join in with worship with any degree of enthusiasm, and she was worried about what others would think about her. Despite this, she believed that people were praying for her, and she was grateful for this. Importantly, her faith was her main reason for not acting on her suicidal ideation. To take her own life would be wrong. 'Christians do not do that kind of thing.'

My conversation with Hannah was not 'spiritual' in the way that my conversation with Sarah implicitly was, and yet we explicitly talked a lot about spirituality and religion. We had a shared, Christian worldview which in some ways may have increased my understanding of her concerns but in other ways presented a danger of possible misunderstandings (as Hannah was concerned there might have been with the chaplain). The important thing that Sarah and I had shared was an experience of how deeply painful life can be. The important thing that Hannah and I shared, at least in its Christian essentials, was a worldview. It was important to Hannah that she should share this worldview with her psychiatrist (or at least *a* psychiatrist) in order that she should feel understood. Actually, I think that the consultant caring for her understood her well and was offering completely appropriate treatment. My only real contribution was to affirm positive religious coping. However, for Hannah, the psychiatrist–patient relationship only adequately encompassed the spiritual domain when she knew that she was speaking to a psychiatrist who shared her spiritual outlook.

A very real question arises as to how far Hannah and I did share a common spiritual outlook. Unlike the chaplain, I had been careful to avoid saying anything specific about my own Christian faith so as to avoid finding myself similarly dismissed, as he had been. I well remember another clinical encounter, many years earlier, where a patient had unexpectedly asked me, in the middle of a consultation and with no warning, 'Are you a Christian?' My answer, in the affirmative, had led to a very unhelpful conversation in which it became clear that he had strongly held views about what Christians think about sexuality and, even though I did not share those views, this led to a breakdown of the therapeutic alliance. (I so wish I had answered 'I wonder why you ask that question?', rather than giving a direct answer!) So, with Hannah, things could also have gone terribly wrong if it had become clear to her that my 'kind' of Christianity was not her own, but the focus here was on her spirituality, not mine.

Patients come to mental health services from all cultural and religious backgrounds. Some may describe themselves as neither spiritual nor religious, but most will come with some sense of spiritual and/or religious identity and with ideas about what that means to them, and how it relates to the particular form of distress that provides the reason for their seeking help. For many, but not all, this will include a belief in God, or gods, or a Higher Power of some kind. Extensive research now shows that these beliefs provide comfort and support during illness and adversity. They also provide a framework of understanding within which conversations about illness and recovery can be had.

Whilst much research on patient preferences for spirituality in mental health care has come from the USA (e.g., Sandage et al., 2020), a key study in the UK was the Somerset

Spirituality Project. Although conducted more than two decades ago, the findings – concerned with the importance of spirituality to service users – remain deeply relevant today. One service user who participated in this qualitative research project, led by a team including service users, said: 'I have had a bad experience with psychiatrists. They will tell me it's all in the mind . . . it's anxiety or depression, and they don't understand what's going on in me . . . many of them have secular ways of thinking. They're not spiritually orientated and they have a very very twisted view of what the church is' (Mental Health Foundation, 2002, p.25). Quotes such as this, and there are many of them in the published findings, reveal just how deep the epistemic divide between psychiatrists and patients can be. It is the task of the psychiatrist not to defend an agnostic or atheistic worldview, which is often only further reinforced by claims that health service delivery is a secular concern, but rather to show an ability to respect, relate to and engage with the spiritual concerns of patients. This does not mean abandoning psychological or biological understandings of mental health but, rather, appreciating them within a holistic context that addresses both the biopsychosocial model and its spiritual and theological concomitants.

Bringing Spirituality Centre Stage

Epstein's conversations with his patients about Buddhism have particular resonance because of the psychological nature of Buddhist philosophy, whether or not any given patient identifies as Buddhist. However, there are also psychological models of spirituality within Christianity, going right back to the teachings of Jesus (Cook, 2020c), through to the sayings of the Desert Fathers and Mothers of the fourth century, and especially evident in Orthodox spirituality (Cook, 2012a), but also in Catholic and Protestant spiritualities of the modern period and in other religions. It is neither necessary nor helpful to impose a pragmatic atheism upon psychiatry, whereby the psychological teachings of the world's major faith traditions are ignored and excluded. Rather, the inherent psychological wisdom of different faith traditions can be utilised in clinical practice to the benefit of patients.

There is now extensive research on the ways in which psychological interventions offered by therapists may take into account religious diversity, seeing this as an asset to treatment rather than as a problem to be overcome (Richards and Bergin, 2000). Spirituality may be effectively integrated into psychotherapy (Pargament, 2011; Rosmarin et al., 2019) and there are spiritual struggles which need to be identified and addressed within treatment (Pargament and Exline, 2022). There is evidence that faith-adapted psychological therapies perform at least as well as standard psychological treatments but with some possible benefits in terms of spiritual outcomes (Worthington et al., 2011; Anderson et al., 2015; Captari et al., 2018).

There has been especially good progress with developing religiously integrated versions of cognitive behavioural therapy (rCBT). In rCBT, teachings of the major faith traditions in relation to thoughts, emotions and behaviours are shown to be consonant with the principles of CBT. Scripture, prayer and other religious resources are then used in support of challenging negative thoughts (Pearce et al., 2014; Koenig et al., 2015; Rosmarin, 2018). Of course, rCBT is not simply CBT repackaged with a religious label. Whilst it shares the same objective of cognitive restructuring, it also incorporates different values, assumptions, narratives and practices than does conventional CBT. For example, in relation to Islam, emphasis on individualism, secularism, self-actualisation and self-expression may be replaced by emphasis on community, interdependence, self-control and spirituality (Husain and Hodge, 2016).

Accepting that there must always be safeguards to protect patients against proselytising and other abuses of spirituality/religion within medicine, the question arises as to how psychiatrists might offer a properly integrated approach to assessment, diagnosis, treatment and recovery, within which spiritualty/religion plays a positive role. A considerable amount of work has been undertaken in relation to assessment (Ross et al., 2022), although there is reason to be concerned that such assessments are still not routinely undertaken in practice. There has been consideration of the ways in which the diagnostic significance of psycho-pathology should be interpreted in relation to religion (Sims, 2016; Cullinan et al., 2024). Integration into treatment has, however, been limited to relatively specific areas, such as rCBT. This may be in part owing to lack of adequate training of psychiatrists, and associated concerns about lack of expertise, or perhaps fears of transgressing professional boundaries in ways that may attract accusations of professional misconduct.

The Spirituality of Patients

In a study of mental health service users in Birmingham, 55 per cent rated spirituality/ religion as either 'very' or 'quite' important to them (Barber et al., 2017). Ratings of the importance of spirituality in surveys in other countries reveal even higher figures. For example, in one US study, 71 per cent of participants reported that spirituality played an important part in their recovery (Bussema and Bussema, 2007). Themes that emerge from qualitative research as spiritually important to mental health patients include such things as meaning-making, identity, spiritual struggles, coping, spiritual impact of symptoms, and relationships (Milner et al., 2020; Barber, 2022).

It is therefore not surprising that patients report, in qualitative research, that they would like spiritual care to be included within mental health care in the UK and elsewhere. In one qualitative study in the UK, respondents reported that a spiritual support group assisted them generally in their subjective sense of mental wellness and also provided a safe space within which they could address their sense of spiritual confusion (Forrester-Jones et al., 2018). In a study in the Netherlands, comparing a Christian clinic and a secular clinic, religious patients in both clinics described negative experiences in relation to a religiosity gap (perceived discordance of spirituality/religion between staff and patients) and positive experiences in relation to a religiosity match (perceived concordance). Patients saw a religiosity match as a precondition for disclosure of spiritual/religious concerns to staff (Van Nieuw Amerongen-Meeuse et al., 2019). These are exactly the concerns that Hannah was sharing when she asked if she could be referred to see me.

In another qualitative study conducted in the Netherlands, outpatients with a diagnosis of bipolar disorder were asked about their spiritual/religious experiences during episodes of mania and depression (Ouwehand et al., 2014, 2018). Participants variously reported, during acute episodes of mania, mystical experiences, visions of angels or intense light, spiritual/religious insights and a sense of divine/spiritual mission. During depressive epi-sodes, fewer religious/spiritual experiences were reported but, where they were mentioned, they involved such things as a sense of the absence of God, absence of meaning, absence of life goals and a sense of emptiness. Some reported a sense of the presence of evil; others experienced feelings of guilt. Despite this, these patients also reported that their faith/ spirituality was a support during their depressive episodes, and that they found religious practices (prayer, meditation, Bible reading, journalling, etc.) helpful. For most participants, whilst acknowledging the medical explanation for their illness, they also believed that their experiences had spiritual/existential significance. Participants expressed a wish that there should be better collaboration between spiritual care staff and mental health professionals during treatment and that a more existential/hermeneutical approach towards religious experiences should be adopted by staff.

The significance of spiritual/religious experiences during illness is only properly appreciated in narrative context (Cook et al., 2016). In conjunction with an understanding of psychiatric phenomenology, narrative provides a key tool in support of making a diagnosis and in gaining a deeper understanding of a patient's concerns. However, a common approach – taking into account the history and mental state examination – has been to try to distinguish between 'genuine' spiritual experiences and psychopathology (see, for example, De Menezes and Moreira-Almeida, 2009). The research undertaken by Ouwehand and her colleagues shows that this is approach is fundamentally flawed. A spiritual experience may be both authentically meaningful, as a spiritual experience, and a manifestation of illness. To deny the spiritual/existential meaning of such experiences represents a form of epistemic injustice, whereby patients are discredited as epistemic agents, and thus not taken seriously as interpreters of their own experiences (Crichton et al., 2017; Cullinan et al., 2024).

Patient-Centred Spirituality

Whilst patient-centred care is increasingly seen as important, there are those who see it as utilitarian and lacking in something significant. It has been suggested that what is really needed is a 'way of being' on the part of the doctor that 'enters into a patient's world of suffering' (Ruiz-Moral, 2022). Others have suggested that being a patient increases physician empathy, and that current medical education actually distances doctors from their patients (Chatterjee, 2012). I think that my own reflections, as I look back on more than 40 years since I qualified as a doctor, lead me to the conclusion that there is no such thing as a 'patient'. Rather, there are only interactions between human beings who come together in the context of suffering, one of whom is professionally identified as a person giving care, and one receiving care. The good doctor, and not least the good psychiatrist, is able to enter into the experience of his or her patient with compassion and genuine concern. Of course, the good psychiatrist also brings professional expertise, experience of working with other patients and all the resources that he or she can muster from the world of modern medicine. However, none of this is likely to matter much if she or he cannot establish the therapeutic alliance that is at the heart of good medicine.

Donald Winnicott, on whose works psychiatrists from diverse spiritualities have drawn, including Frank Lake and Mark Epstein, once said that there is 'no such thing as an infant', by which he meant that 'whenever one finds an infant one finds maternal care, and without maternal care there would be no infant' (Winnicott, 1982, p.39). It might similarly be said that 'there is no such thing as a patient' (Casher, 2013). That is, wherever one finds a patient, one finds medical care, and without medical care there would be no patient. Having said this, a number of caveats immediately need to be affirmed. Medical care must be considered broadly, and includes all the allied healthcare professions, including psychology and psychotherapy, and not just medicine and nursing. The risk of infantilisation of patients is also very real and, although regression may to some extent be inevitable, the proper aim will always be to foster autonomy and maturity. The psychiatrist–patient relationship is (leaving aside for a moment child and adolescent psychiatry) a relationship between two adults, one of whom comes to the other seeking help in the context of suffering. This delicate relationship is vulnerable to abuses of power, including the abuse of medical privilege as an opportunity to proselytise. However, at its best, it encompasses empathy, compassion and a common humanity, within which each psychiatrist will have her (or his) own way of being, enabling her to stand alongside her patients in their suffering as a basis for offering what help she can. Spirituality plays a central part in this process, whether named as such or not, sharing with psychiatry a capacity to create transitional space. Within such transitional spaces the human capacities to construct narrative, reflect on meaning and find a pathway to recovery in the face of suffering, chaos and uncertainty can be fostered.

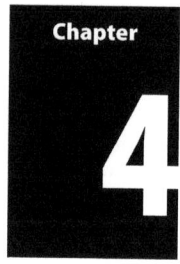

Psychiatry and Theology

The religiosity gap between clinicians and patients in mental health services expresses itself in a variety of ways. For example, I have all too frequently heard it said by patients that 'my clinician does not understand my faith . . . he says it is a part of the illness'. I have been asked (usually by email) to confirm, for the benefit of unbelieving clinicians, that a patient's experiences are 'from God' and not a part of their illness. When I was a relatively new consultant, a psychologist (who obviously didn't know me very well) said in our multidisciplinary team meeting that a particular patient's problems 'would be resolved if only she gave up her Catholic faith'. Clinicians, on the other hand, often find it difficult to talk about God with their patients, for fear of crossing professional boundaries (which will be discussed further in Chapter 8).

The gap between individual patients and clinicians is not the only problem. There is a fundamental problem with the way in which mental health services in the UK (and not only in the UK) deal with spirituality and religion. The starting point seems to be with a view that reflects much more the perspectives of Freud, or at best Maudsley, rather than those of Jung, Lake or Epstein. Religion is, somewhere within the structures of mental health service delivery, seen as at best irrelevant (but tolerated for those who find it helpful) and at worst a part of the problem. Spirituality, in a generic sense, fares a little better but is still seen as an optional extra.

This perspective is rarely articulated explicitly, unless sometimes in unguarded comments like those of the psychologist in my multidisciplinary team, or perhaps in the rhetoric of the National Secular Society (Sanchez, 2023). It is also true that chaplains are available in most (but not all) NHS trusts, albeit only in small numbers, reflecting an assumption that most patients will not need to see them. All the main psychological and pharmacological treatment options are offered without reference to spirituality or religion, and – as such – are assumed to be an adequate provision. In this way, a pragmatic atheism is closely entangled with mental health service provision. Until recently, this has been reflected in training of mental health professionals, which gives no attention to matters of spirituality, theology or religion, except perhaps – in passing – in transcultural psychiatry. Some NHS trusts have dispensed with chaplaincy/spiritual care completely.

In correspondence published in *Psychiatric Bulletin* in 2008, Professor Rob Poole described psychiatrists as 'essentially applied biopsychosocial scientists'. I disagree with this, given that I think psychiatry has much to learn from the humanities as well as the sciences (Bhugra and Ventriglio, 2015; Datta, 2016; Oyebode, 2018). The scientific status of psychiatry is also contested by proponents of critical psychiatry (Thomas and Bracken, 2018) and, although I obviously don't agree with them, we need to be careful not to fall into the trap of arguing for the benefits of psychiatry on primarily scientific grounds. Scientific expertise is not necessarily what patients value most (McCarthy, 2014; Murphy, 2024). However, Poole's statement does reflect an important point of view. Whilst patients want their doctors to have 'a good bedside manner', modern medicine is fundamentally evidence based, and the 'evidence' is usually provided by science.

As a science, psychiatry is highly interdisciplinary, drawing on the social sciences as well as the natural sciences. Neuroscience offers a vision by way of which, so some are persuaded, it may one day identify the scientific foundations of all mental disorders (Kirmayer and Crafa, 2014). However, the widespread acceptance of the biopsychosocial model (Engel, 1977) acknowledges that biology alone offers a reductionist perspective and that the psychological and social dimensions of the human condition are important to a complete understanding of health and disease. This raises difficult questions about the ways in which causality operates across different – biological, psychological, social – levels of the model (Stoyanov et al., 2013; De Haan, 2021), especially concerning interactions between mind and brain (Glannon, 2020).

Strangely enough, it is in the domain of scientific research that arguments in support of giving more attention to spirituality/religion in psychiatry have gained most ground in recent decades (Koenig and Larson, 2001; Koenig et al., 2024). Criticisms of this research have emerged from theology and the humanities, as well as within the medical and scientific community, but the premise that science provides evidence for the benefits of spirituality/religion, rather than against it, is radically different from anything that Maudsley or Freud expected. This has led to arguments from some quarters that the three-level biopsychosocial model is insufficient and should be replaced by a biopsychosocial-spiritual model (Hiatt, 1986; Kuhn, 1988). This, of course, only further complexifies the debate about how these different levels can be understood as interrelating causally, conceptually and ontologically. How, then, can we understand the relationship between spirituality and the biopsychosocial model?

Theology

Spirituality and religion are, like psychiatry, highly interdisciplinary fields of study, drawing broadly upon the social sciences, as well as the humanities. After the scientific paradigm, 'study of religion' and 'religious studies' adopt more objectifying perspectives. Theology, on the other hand, tends to be more confessional and associated with a first-person perspective. This is not to say that it cannot be academically critical and, to confuse things further, there is much interest in 'empirical theology' and the adoption of scientific methods in order to further theological understanding. However, it is easier to distinguish 'being religious' from study of religion than it is to distinguish it from theology. There is no 'view from nowhere' and all study of theology and religion is humanly situated and contextual.

Theology has many 'voices'. Helen Cameron et al. (2010) identify four: normative (official teachings such as creeds and doctrines); formal (academic theology, and theology in dialogue with other disciplines); espoused (as articulated by a given group); and operant (as implicitly embedded in practice). Whilst formal theology is the natural academic dialogue partner with psychiatry, the other three voices may sometimes be important in research. For example, normative and espoused theologies of sexuality and gender may contribute to the mental health burden experienced by LGBTQ people, or operant theologies of forgiveness may impact upon the outcomes of forgiveness therapy, and such relationships are all amenable to empirical research. All of these voices may therefore be important in research, but the voices that I would suggest are most important to clinical practice are those of 'ordinary' theology.

Ordinary theology (Astley and Francis, 2013) refers to the 'theology and theologizing of Christians who have received little or no theological education of a scholarly, academic or systematic kind' (p.56). I see no reason in principle why we should not also talk of the ordinary theology of adherents to other religions: Islam, Judaism, Hinduism and so on. What matters for most patients, and most psychiatrists, is not what they are supposed to believe (although normative theology is important) but rather what they *do* believe. Ordinary theology is contextual. It is forged in the crucible of human experience and contributes to personal identity and meaning-making. It shapes the various kinds of religiosity that are measured as independent variables in scientific research on spirituality/religion and mental health. More importantly for clinical practice, it reveals itself in the content of psychopathology and shapes personal insight into the causes and significance of mental distress.

For the purposes of this chapter, theology will be considered as 'the intellectual study of the religious dimension of personal experience' (Polkinghorne, 2000, p.19), including experiences of psychopathology. Within this domain of study, as physicist and theologian John Polkinghorne points out, 'atheism is a possible theological option' (p.19). There is therefore no presumption, a priori, concerning the superiority of any particular theology over another, except insofar as the ordinary theologies of patients must be respected within patient-centred care. There is, however, a recognition that theology, as Tom McLeish (another physicist) has argued, is concerned with 'persons, communities, relationships, living experienced stories … Because theology observes and construes stories, it is able to discuss purposes and values – it can speak of, and ground "teleology"' (McLeish, 2014, p.214).

The good psychiatrist facilitates the telling of stories by patients. Patients usually want to tell their story to their clinicians. For the patient, this exercise is, at least in part, a search for meaning and purpose, although that search might take many different forms and words like 'God' or 'spirituality' will often not be mentioned. Both psychiatrist and patient come to the encounter with a set of values (which may or may not coincide). For the psychiatrist, understanding the meanings, purposes and values embedded in their patients' stories is a key part of patient-centred practice. The Royal College of Psychiatrists (2017) has its own *Core Values for Psychiatrists*, which include some very spiritual qualities, such as humility and honesty. However, psychiatry is also about discovering what patients value and working with their values (as much as possible) in a patient-centred fashion. In this way, at least if we adopt McLeish's understanding of theology, both psychiatrists and patients are, usually without realising it, doing theology all the time.

Science

There is now an extensive evidence base concerned with the scientific study of spirituality/religion and mental health. Religiosity correlates with better mental health, at least in relation to depression and substance misuse, and probably also in relation to dementia and stress-related disorders. It is associated with lower rates of suicide (Bonelli and Koenig, 2013; Koenig et al., 2020b). The evidence in relation to anxiety disorders is more mixed and there appears to be no association in relation to major mental health disorders such as schizophrenia and bipolar disorder. Spiritual struggles of various kinds can have an adverse impact on mental health and may sometimes need to be the focus of therapy (Martínez De Pisón, 2022; Pargament and Exline, 2022). Much of the research has been cross-sectional and is not able to demonstrate causal relationships.

A recent meta-analysis of 48 longitudinal studies showed a relationship between religiosity and mental health in relation to only two out of eight measures of spirituality/religion: participation in public religious activities and importance of religion. Effect sizes were small (Garssen et al., 2020). Meta-analyses have their limitations, for example in relation to heterogeneity of subject samples, methodology and effect sizes of the studies included, and this particular meta-analysis focussed on 'emotional health', rather than on mental disorders (Koenig et al., 2020a). This is therefore far from the last word on the scientific research, and it is to be hoped that future research, and future meta-analyses, will shed further light on the complex relationships between spirituality/religion and mental health. However, the headline findings, interpreted by those so inclined as 'religion is good for you', and by those otherwise inclined as of questionable significance, are only a part of the story.

Much of the research to date has focussed on independent variables which are easy to measure, such as participation in religious activities (public or private). This does not take into account the motivation for such activities. An early paper by Gordon Allport and Michael Ross (1967) demonstrated an important distinction between two fundamental kinds of religious orientation. Intrinsic religiosity is concerned with religion as a central guiding motivation in life. Extrinsic religiosity is concerned with social and personal utility of religious practice. Subsequent research has shown that intrinsic, but not extrinsic, religiosity is associated with better mental health (Mahmoodabad et al., 2016). The overall associations between religiosity and mental health may therefore hide within group differences between differently motivated groups of religious subjects.

Initially, both intrinsic and extrinsic religiosity were conceptualised as dimensional constructs, each on a spectrum from weak to strong motivation. However, it soon became clear that this was too simple, that there might be confounding variables and that the causal relationships were impossible to work out from largely cross-sectional studies. The dichotomy is also patently judgemental, with 'intrinsic' implicitly evaluated as good, and 'extrinsic' as bad. Although the general association with mental health has remained in subsequent research, many inconsistent studies have been reported and it has become clear that there are cultural, religious and other factors which influence the findings (Park, 2021). Intrinsic religiosity is probably better viewed as a measure of religious commitment, whereas extrinsic religiosity measures 'the sort of religion that gives religion a bad name' (Donahue, 1985). Later, C. Daniel Batson (1976) proposed a third motivational construct, that of religion as 'quest'. Those who adopt a questing approach to religion are constantly questioning and seeking in response to the challenges that life inevitably throws up, both for the individual and for wider society.

The research on religious motivation is thus a cautionary tale, warning against premature or simplistic conclusions based upon inadequate methodologies or false assumptions. Behind the independent variables that are operationalised within research there may well lie complex (and often mixed) motivations for religious affiliation and spiritual practices.

Qualitative research also has its part to play, especially in relation to understanding the needs and concerns of patients and thus in clarifying the nature of the religiosity gap between mental health professionals and their patients. In one recent review of 38 qualitative studies across 15 countries, six key themes emerged that were identified as important to people experiencing 'mental health difficulties' (Milner et al., 2020). These were:

meaning-making, identity, service provision, being able to talk with staff about their difficulties in spiritual/religious terms, the relationship between spirituality and mental health symptoms, and spiritual coping. Amongst these themes, spiritual/religious coping may be especially important.

Religious coping is employed by people of diverse ethnicity, from different religious traditions and with no formal religious affiliation, as a means of coping with mental distress (Bhui et al., 2009). Methods of religious coping are diverse and involve both cognitive appraisals and coping activities (Pargament et al., 1990). In an early paper, Pargament et al. (1988) identified three styles of coping: collaborative (working together with God), deferring (in which the individual looks to God for help/answers) and self-directing (an active coping style, emphasising human agency). Wong-McDonald and Gorsuch (2000) later identified a fourth style, named surrender, in which an active choice is made to surrender to God's will.[1] The collaborative style has generally been associated with positive outcomes. The deferring and self-directing styles have demonstrated somewhat mixed results in research (Yangarber-Hicks, 2004).

Two broad kinds of religious coping have been identified (Pargament et al., 1998). Positive religious coping includes such things as seeking support and help from, and closer connection with, God, seeking to work together with God, reappraising circumstances in terms of God's good purposes ('benevolent' reappraisals), seeking and giving forgiveness, and refocussing attention on religious concerns. Negative religious coping includes such things as interpreting circumstances as God's punishment, doubting God, questioning God's love and care, questioning the intentions of the faith community, and various interpretations of events as owing to demonic/evil influence. Positive religious coping has been associated with good mental adjustment and negative religious coping with poor mental health outcomes.

Negative religious coping may be associated with spiritual struggles concerning the tensions, conflicts and distress associated with spiritual/religious issues (Exline and Rose, 2013). Negative religious coping and spiritual struggles are not exactly the same thing, and some people may engage in the former without experiencing the latter (Pirutinsky, 2024), but they are similarly associated with poorer psychological adjustment (Bockrath et al., 2022; Cowden et al., 2022), may impact on medical mortality (Pargament et al., 2001) and may result in changing theological views of the nature of God (Van Tongeren et al., 2019). Outcomes are not necessarily negative and spiritual struggles may lead to post-traumatic growth (Stauner et al., 2020). Spiritual struggles are experienced by those who identify as spiritual but not religious (SBNR) and by those who are religiously unaffiliated, as well as by those who self-identify as religious (Mercadante, 2020).

The Religious and Spiritual Struggles Scale, developed by Julie Exline et al. (2014), identifies six domains of struggle: divine (negative emotional associations with God), demonic (attributions of events/experiences to evil spiritual forces), interpersonal (related to religious people/institutions), moral (ethical dilemmas or guilt), doubt (in relation to faith) and ultimate meaning (lack of meaning in life). The scale demonstrated good reliability and validity in the original, American and largely Christian, subject sample. As

---

[1] Although a factor analysis identified this as a separate style, it seems to draw conceptually on both deferring and collaborative styles, and is built upon a specifically Christian theological premise. It has been used in some subsequent research (Clements and Ermakova, 2012), but generally appears to have been less widely adopted in research.

the authors acknowledge, it would need adaptation for other contexts, especially in relation to polytheistic religions and non-religious spiritualities.

Research also shows that a range of spiritual interventions for various mental disorders are associated with good outcomes. These include 12-step facilitation, mindfulness, compassion-focussed therapy, religiously integrated cognitive behavioural therapy (CBT), forgiveness therapy, spiritually integrated interventions for survivors of sexual abuse, spiritually integrated cognitive processing therapy and a range of other spiritually integrated approaches to psychotherapy (Cook and Powell, 2022, pp.249–292; see also Chapter 7, this volume).

Until recently, little research had been undertaken in relation to the so-called nones, that is, those who answer 'none of the above' in questionnaires about religious affiliation. People who do not identify with any particular religion are far from being a homogenous group. Atheists, agnostics and the SBNR may all have very different relationships with mental health and well-being. Some recent research suggests that, in fact, atheists may have similar mental health to those who identify as religious (Moore and Leach, 2016; Baker et al., 2018). In a systematic review of 14 studies (Weber et al., 2012), greater certainty in belief, whether in religion or atheism, was associated with better psychological health. Other studies have found a curvilinear relationship with mental health, although the nature of the relationship varies between studies. For example, in one US study there was a curvilinear relationship between mental well-being and certainty of belief, so that those with a higher certainty (whether religious or atheist) had better mental well-being than those with low certainty (including agnostics and those who are unsure) (Galen and Kloet, 2010).

Overall, however, it is not clear that the findings of research consistently support this analysis of the equal benefits of certainty, whether in relation to belief or unbelief. In a Brazilian study (Gontijo et al., 2022), the curvilinear relationship was more complex, with spiritual beliefs predicting only meaning in life (not mental health) and religious/spiritual experiences being differently related to positive and negative definitions of mental health. In one US study, psychological well-being was actually poorer amongst atheists and agnostics than amongst those with religious affiliation and those with no religious preference (Hayward et al., 2016). In another Brazilian study (Vitorino et al., 2018), those who might be described as SBNR (high spirituality but low religiousness) were happier but also more anxious than those low in both spirituality and religiousness.

Aside from methodological differences between studies (which may be significant), the context of belief/non-belief may be important, with very different cultural and religious environments between some studies (e.g., Brazil is not the same as the USA). In one US study of adolescents, in which non-religious teens had higher overall rates of mental illness, those at greatest disadvantage were the non-religious whose parents were both highly religious (Kugelmass and Garcia, 2015).

Science and Theology in Psychiatry

Ian Barbour (1998) proposed four basic ways of relating science and religion: conflict, independence, dialogue and integration. Whilst some ways of relating might overlap categories, this is a generally useful way of looking at interactions between science and theology/religion.

Barbour's examples of conflict included the stories of Galileo and Darwin, both popularly perceived as battles taking place within 'the warfare between science and religion'. Both stories are more complex than popularly understood, but Darwin's story is particularly relevant here. In his book *On the Origin of Species* (1859), Charles Darwin (1809–1882) proposed that the diversity of the biological order had come about, across many thousands of years, as living organisms adapted to their environments through a process of natural selection operating upon inherited variation. This was not hugely controversial at the time insofar as the Christian churches were concerned. However, it has come into conflict with some more recent literalist interpretations of the book of Genesis and has thus become a point of contention for some Christians and others.[2]

Barbour's model of independence is one of 'totally independent and autonomous' enterprises (Barbour, 1998, p.84). This is perhaps best illustrated by the subsequent work of Stephen J. Gould (1999), who proposed that science and religion represent non-overlapping magisteria (NOMA). The 'magisterium' (domain of teaching) of science addresses the empirical order, whereas the magisterium of religion is concerned with such things as ultimate meaning and ethics. The two domains, or magisteria, are not in conflict because they are simply talking about different things.

The model of dialogue, according to Barbour, addresses areas of common concern between science and theology by way of conversation. In such dialogues, theology may challenge the more reductionist perspectives of science, and science might raise important questions for theology. Popular topics for dialogue have included cosmology, creation/evolution and – notably for our purposes here – the relationship between mind and body, and theological anthropology.

Finally, the model of integration attempts to provide a unified scientific and theological account. Barbour describes three variations on this approach: natural theology, a theology of nature and systematic synthesis. Examples include, respectively, natural theological discussions of the anthropic principle (the way in which the universe appears to be 'fine-tuned' for the possibility of life), the work of Teilhard de Chardin integrating Christian theology and evolution, and the process philosophy of Alfred North Whitehead (1861–1947) in which a very different understanding of God emerges from that of the major monotheistic religions.

All four of these models have relevance to spirituality/religion in psychiatry. Barbour's model of conflict operates on a theological spectrum from scientific materialism at the one end to biblical literalism at the other. Scientific materialism within psychiatry may express itself in some interpretations of evolutionary psychiatry (Flannelly et al., 2010; Phillips et al., 2020). Neuroscientific accounts of religion and religious experience may follow a reductionistic trajectory, understanding experiences of God as generated within the limbic system, or else it may be argued that it is inevitable that human experiences of the transcendent, however one understands a transcendent reality, must at some point register as measurable changes in the brain (Phillips et al., 2020). At the other end of the spectrum, there are those who reject psychiatry because of their religious beliefs. Extreme religious movements such as scientology see psychiatry as completely opposed to (their) religion (McCall, 2006). Some subgroups within mainstream religion take a not dissimilar stance. For example, the biblical counselling movement, formerly known as nouthetic counselling, originated in the work of Jay Adams (1929–2020), an American Presbyterian pastor who was influenced by the work of Thomas Szasz. Nouthetic counselling emphasised personal responsibility and human sinfulness and promoted use of the Bible as the primary text for

---

[2] For some helpful reviews from a Christian perspective, see Edwards, 1999 and Berry, 2007.

pastoral care. It was characterised by a marked distrust of psychiatry and psychology (Kinghorn, 2016). At a somewhat less extreme location on the spectrum, there are many worldwide whose negative attitudes to psychiatry are associated with strong religious beliefs (Zieger et al., 2017; Ta et al., 2018) and others for whom specific issues may pose a barrier to seeking help from mental health professionals (e.g., in relation to jinn/spirits/demons as perceived causes of mental ill health – see Chapter 6).

It might be argued that the existing model of healthcare delivery in the UK is an example of NOMA of science/medicine and religion/spiritual care. This is not completely true, and things may be better in some of the devolved nations (Kelly, 2012), and in some NHS trusts in England, than in others. Nonetheless spiritual care is delivered by a separate group of professionals (chaplains) who are not fully integrated into the multidisciplinary team in most NHS mental health services. Every patient gets to see a nurse and/or a doctor, but the vast majority do not get to see a chaplain; confidentiality may impede communication between the chaplain and the clinical team; and record-keeping is often separate. Of course, things do not need to be this way and Koenig writes of initiatives in the USA that seek a fuller integration of spirituality into patient care (Koenig, 2014).

A degree of research dialogue between spirituality/religion and psychiatry is evidenced by the now huge literature on spirituality, religion and mental health (e.g., Koenig, 2018; Cook and Powell, 2022), albeit this is more scientific than theological in emphasis. Clinical dialogue is evidenced in service developments (Cook et al., 2012), in the running of spiritual support groups (Forrester-Jones et al., 2018) and in the development of spiritually integrated therapies (see Chapter 8). Neurotheology, a field of study barely two decades old, 'linking the neurosciences with religion and theology', aspires to offer a 'two way street' for interdisciplinary dialogue (Newberg, 2010, p.45).[3] However, certain kinds of dialogue still seem to be rare. The dialogue between formal theology and psychiatry is still largely restricted to Christian theology (Cook, 2023b). Interfaith dialogue on mental health is surprisingly limited, although the Mental Health and Faith Community Partnership, involving a collaboration of the American Association of People with Disabilities and the American Psychiatric Association, provides a good model of how to develop resources to train both religious leaders and psychiatrists in such a way as to support recovery from mental illness (Ramsey-Lucas, 2016).

Integration of theology/spirituality and psychiatry, to a greater or lesser extent, is always likely to be the quest in the mind of the individual psychiatrist. Of the psychiatrists considered in Chapter 2, Freud, and to a lesser extent Maudsley, adopted a conflictual way of relating to religion. The others variously developed an integrative model. Jung, Epstein and Lake reflected on religion and clinical practice over many years, leading each to their own systematically unified understanding. In Jung's case, this was across religious traditions, although predominantly influenced by Christianity, whereas in Epstein's writings and Lake's *Clinical Theology* there is an attempt to integrate psychoanalytic thinking

---

[3] In practice this can sometimes seem like a one-way street. For example, although talking about 'shared areas of concern' and how 'each worldview can and should inform and enrich the other', one review (Klemm, 2019, p.1) finds that neuroscience 'help[s] us understand why we believe certain religious ideas and not others', 'explains our behavior and might even help us live more righteous and fulfilled lives', and leads to 'religious perspectives that are more reasoned, mature, satisfying, and beneficial'. Religion, on the other hand, seems only to point to 'areas of religious debate that that scientific research might help resolve'.

with, respectively, Buddhism and Christianity. Kharitidi's books offer an autobiographical account of her personal journey as a psychiatrist who absorbed experiences of shamanism, but do not evidence the same level of theoretical integration. To some extent this book is my own attempt at integration, although it also includes dialogue, and I am attempting to address integration across different traditions of faith and spirituality, rather than within a particular tradition. I would write it differently if I were addressing a narrowly Christian readership, but not very differently. My clinical theology would look very different from that of Frank Lake (1966). For example, my approach is less about psychoanalysis than his was, and more about spirituality as integral to the biopsychosocial model in psychiatry. I would take a different approach to managing the theological balance between scripture, tradition and reason.

Integration, in the mind of the psychiatrist, is always likely to be about eliminating or avoiding the cognitive dissonance that unintegrated mental models of theology and psychiatry might otherwise bring. It is therefore likely to be very individualistic. Integration in wider professional and theological contexts must inevitably return to dialogue as different psychiatrists (even if they share a faith tradition) are likely to have different views on how to go about integration.

Looking at things somewhat differently, we might say that Freud, as the individual psychiatrist, developed an integration of atheism with psychiatry. The danger is that atheism is considered as the default, or 'neutral', starting point and is not seen as a theological perspective. It is in fact not a position of neutrality and is perceived by many patients as deeply unsympathetic to religion. The inner psyche of Freud the man, I might dare suggest, was seeking integration. The professional and intellectual engagement of Freud in dialogue with others was highly conflictual.

Formal Dialogue

Scientific research showing a positive relationship between spirituality/religion and mental health may seem to be very theologically attractive. However, on closer examination, the way in which scientific research findings have typically been received and understood presents significant theological problems.

In *Heal Thyself*, Joel Shuman and Keith Meador (2003) systematically examine scientific research in a theological context. Although they write from the perspective of Christian theology, much of what they have to say has wider relevance. A particular concern that they raise relates to the difference between a patient-centred understanding of spirituality/religion as an important part of what makes a person who she is, and a utilitarian approach to advocating spirituality/religion to a patient in order to improve their health and well-being.

Religions are traditionally concerned not primarily with health but with 'living and dying faithfully'. Shuman and Meador suggest that this means 'living and dying in harmony with the deity, with other persons, and with the rest of the world – whether in sickness or in health' (Shuman and Meador, 2003, p.21). Most of the scientific research, in contrast, takes a generic approach to religion, assuming some kind of common 'core' according to which differences amongst religious traditions are not significant, at least not in terms of health outcomes. So, the truthfulness of what is believed does not matter so much as that you believe. This corresponds to what George Lindbeck (2009) refers to as the 'experiential-expressive' model of religion, which 'interprets doctrines as non-informative and non-discursive symbols of inner feelings, attitudes, or existential orientations' (p.2). Religion (or spirituality) thus conceived is a highly individualistic affair. This contrasts with religion more traditionally understood as offering that which 'molds and shapes the self and its world, rather than [being] an expression or thematization of a preexisting self or of preconceptual experience' (Lindbeck, 2009, p.20). The experiential-expressive religion implicit within scientific research is not the particular kind of religion lived by most patients (although it may correspond to some forms of non-religious spirituality); rather, according to Shuman and Meador, it is a 'vaguely defined and nontraditional' religion, 'with its own particular account of the ends of human life and its own implicit doctrine of God, humanity, and the rest of creation' (p.40):

> The most significant theological question about the interrelationship of religion and health is not simply whether being more religious will result in better health but whether the religion in question, that is, the religion that ostensibly improves the health of some, teaches its adherents the sometimes difficult truth about God and God's creation and helps them live well in and as part of that creation – whether they are sick or well. And this is not an empirical but a theological question. (Shuman and Meador, 2003, p.45)

The situation as Shuman and Meador describe it in North America (and much of their account applies to Europe as well) is further compounded by what they refer to as the advent of the 'therapeutic culture' of consumer society. In a therapeutic culture, 'therapy appears to have become a replacement for religion', within which psychiatrists (and also psychologists, therapists and social workers) emerge as the new 'priestly class' (Shuman and Meador, 2003, p.80). Freud is identified as a key theorist in the early days of this movement, a movement which has now influenced many faith communities as they focus on how to meet people's needs. In this context, health is commodified, and God becomes 'useful' and controllable for the end of obtaining health. The central Christian theological affirmations that God is present amidst suffering and that Christians are called to live for God in relationship with others, especially those who suffer, are exchanged for an individualised version of a faith which serves 'me'. Such a view of religion is a serious distortion, not only of Christianity but of all of the religious traditions that are influenced by the same therapeutic culture and consumer society.

In *Selling Spirituality*, Jeremy Carrette and Richard King (2005) have examined the commodification of spirituality and its 'takeover' from religion in a consumer society. They examine the adverse impact of this process in the reinterpretation of Asian religions such as Taoism, Buddhism and Hinduism. Whereas these traditions, in their authentic and historical forms, offer a critique of consumerism and individualism, their practices have now been privatised and commodified in the secular West, often in the guise of New Age spirituality, to serve the ends of longevity, physical health, stress reduction and personal happiness. Thus, for example, the Hindu practice of yoga in its original context seeks to bring about a cessation of 'mental fluctuations' by eradicating selfish desires. The eventual aim in view is realisation of the true self and liberation from cycles of reincarnation.[4] The secularised view, in contrast, emphasises either physical or mental well-being rather than spiritual well-being. In each case, the original spiritual and theological context is stripped away.

Koenig (2008a) has observed that spirituality is a difficult independent variable to operationalise in research because it is inherently confounded with psychological variables,

---

[4] This is in contrast to Buddhism, which rejects any notion of an enduring 'self'.

and that research should therefore focus more on religion. Unfortunately, scientific research on religion and health has generally not engaged with insights from the humanities and has therefore not recognised that religion is equally difficult to define. Future research needs to be much more interdisciplinary, to engage more critically with these research variables and to move beyond crude measures such as frequency of attendance at religious services. There is also scope for theological research to engage at greater depth with the science of psychiatry. Research on the theology of mental health has been relatively limited and largely confined to the Judeo-Christian tradition (Cook, 2023b).

Ordinary Theology in Psychiatry

Because theology is generally neglected by psychiatry, it is rare to find theological variables explicitly addressed in psychiatric research, except in very basic terms such as belief (or non-belief) in God. The concept of ordinary theology has not yet been applied in psychiatric research or in relation to mental health. In empirical theological research it has usually been adopted within a qualitative research design, and has focussed on specific themes such as prayer requests (Burton, 2015), sacraments (Neil, 2015) or sin (Wright, 2014). However, it has much to offer to research in psychiatry. Just one theme of interest to theology will be considered here, that of psychological representations and theological concepts of God.

God Images

God images are defined in empirical psychological research in terms of 'internal working models of a specific divine attachment figure' and, in principle, are applicable across diverse faith traditions (Davis et al., 2013). God images operate at an 'emotional, physiological, largely nonverbal, and usually implicit level' (Davis et al., 2013, p.52). They are triggered by learnt responses to interpersonal and situational cues and operate in a reflexive and largely unconscious manner (Davis et al., 2013). They thus share key characteristics of ordinary theology, which is also learnt and also has an affective component. Ordinary theology is usually understood as consciously reflected upon; however, it is also 'covert', or 'subterranean', even if not unconscious (Astley and Francis, 2013, pp.70–72). God images thus share some key features with ordinary theology.

Following a view originating with the work of Ana-María Rizzuto, God concept is defined in contrast to God images as 'a person's theological set of beliefs about a specific divine attachment figure's traits; about how that divine attachment figure relates with, thinks about, and feels toward humans (including the self); and about how humans (including the self) should relate with, think about, and feel toward the divine attachment figure' (Davis et al., 2013, p.52). However, not all researchers make such a clear distinction. For example, Schaap-Jonker et al. (2008) take a broader view, in which God image (here synonymous with 'God representation')

> comprises one's emotional understanding of God, which reflects subjective experiences of God and is developed through a relational, and initially unconscious, process in which parents and significant others play a part. Simultaneously, it contains one's cognitive understanding of God, namely the rational, more objective part of the God representation, which is based on what a person learns about God in propositional terms, which in turn is related to the doctrines that are taught and found within the family and the (local) religious culture. (pp.502–503)

God concept, and in its broader usage also God image, may thus be understood as a kind of ordinary theology of the nature of God as a relational object. In an interesting study by Barrett and Keil (1996), it was found that a person may hold multiple God concepts, that there is a tendency to anthropomorphise God and that anthropomorphised God concepts may conflict with theologically abstract God concepts.

God image has been related to mental health in a wide range of studies, perhaps unsurprisingly showing that positive God image is usually related to better mental health (Schaap-Jonker et al., 2002; Greenway et al., 2003; Jonker et al., 2008; Khaksari and Khosravi, 2011; Koohsar and Bonab, 2011a, 2011b; Silton et al., 2014). God image may mediate the relationship between God concept and mental well-being (Hart et al., 2024).

In a US questionnaire study (Bradshaw et al., 2008) involving 1,629 predominantly Christian participants, a perception of God as loving was inversely associated with psychopathology, whereas a perception of God as remote was positively associated with mental health problems. Prayer frequency was positively associated with symptoms, especially amongst those who viewed God as remote, suggesting that people pray more when distressed. However, in a later study (Bradshaw et al., 2010), the same research group found that the link between God image and distress was related to attachment to God. Secure attachment was inversely related to distress and anxious attachment was positively related. Once this was controlled for, there were no net effects of God image on distress. A similar mediating role for God representations has been demonstrated by Tung et al. (2017).

In another US study (Currier et al., 2017) involving 241 predominantly Christian participants in a 'spiritually integrative inpatient programme', pre-treatment God image predicted post-treatment affective status. This effect was mediated by 'religious comforts and strains', including (positively) 'feeling loved by God' and 'beliefs give you a sense of meaning and purpose', and negatively such things as feeling 'abandoned by God' or feeling excessively guilty for sins/mistakes.

In theory, the construct(s) of God image/God concept work across theological traditions. However, Islam traditionally has a concern about the idea of 'images' which might make this problematic for some Muslim research subjects (Rifai, 2019) and there is some evidence to suggest that Hindus may employ images of God differently from Christians and Muslims (Leach et al., 2001).

Clinical Theology

There are various examples of how God images come to the fore in psychotherapy in Frank Lake's *Clinical Theology*. For example, he describes analysis of a priest whose images of God, revealed under LSD abreaction, were 'vague, dark and meaningless' (Lake, 1966, p.636) and 'God the Destroyer' (p.637). The analysis as reported by Lake was incomplete and only partially successful. Perhaps a better example arises from Chris MacKenna's work as a Jungian analyst, where he describes work with a patient whose image of an 'examiner God', a composite of maternal and paternal images, was gradually replaced by a 'beloved', adorable God. For MacKenna (2002), self-images and God images are closely related. The danger is that these images become frozen in time, with correspondingly restrictive consequences for faith and personal development. Ideally, they grow and evolve: 'As our psychological-cum-spiritual development progresses, so our internal God image has to grow and change. In the process, it provides us with an evolving glimpse of a greater unity in which the contradictions of our present existence are somehow encompassed and transcended' (MacKenna, 2002, p.332).

God images are important for both psychiatrists and their patients. In Chapter 2, in relating my experiences of formation as a psychiatrist, I was implicitly charting the evolution of my own images of God as they were challenged and tested by life experience, reading, clinical practice and theological reflection. As a result, I now adopt a much more apophatic spirituality and my God concepts are much more informed by mystical theologies of various kinds, and by a willingness to acknowledge that there is much that I do not know (a kind of negative capability). At the same time, I have found the positive themes of the Christian story, especially in relation to the encounter with God in Christ, to be more (not less) meaningful and life-enriching. In finding deeper theological roots in the Christian tradition, I have found myself more open to, and curious about, the images and concepts of God that I encounter in others (including their atheological images and concepts).

In clinical practice, in working with my patients, God images have arisen as important mainly in two contexts. Firstly, images of God become evident in psychopathology. As such, they tell us about our patients, what is important to them and how they understand God. For example, I remember a Catholic patient who had a diagnosis of bipolar disorder, and when acutely unwell experienced visions of hell, reflecting images of an angry and judgemental God. In theory, her religiosity might have been a protective factor, but negative religious coping (as discussed earlier) tends to be associated with poor mental health outcomes. Sadly, she died by suicide. Another patient, during an acute episode of psychosis, took great delight in telling me that she had gained insights into the nature of God through the image of a mussel. God, she said, is a trinity, just as the mussel has three parts – two halves of a shell and an inner fleshy part. There was no obviously profound insight here, as far as I could see, but it reflected her ordinary theology, and she seemed to enjoy the fact that she could see why it was important even though I could not. If not an example of positive coping, it was at least not unhelpful. She went on to make a good recovery,

Secondly, God images and God concepts were sometimes very important in my work as an addiction psychiatrist. With hindsight, I wish that I had asked patients more often about their images and concepts of God, but it was only later in my career that I became aware of how important they might be for some patients' recovery. In the 12-step programme of Alcoholics Anonymous, and its sister organisations, reference is made to the 'Higher Power', referred to in Step 2 as 'a Power greater than ourselves' and in Steps 3, 5, 6 and 11, explicitly, as 'God'. Despite the wording of these steps, members of AA are not required to believe in God, and they conceive of their Higher Power in a variety of ways. In one survey of 450 members of Narcotics Anonymous in California, 45 per cent reported that they believed in 'God per se' and 36 per cent in a 'universal spirit' (Galanter et al., 2020). In a study of 100 abstinent members of 12-step programmes in the UK, Wendy Dossett (2015) reports on examples of the Higher Power as 'an ongoing creativity which is infinite'(p.28), a feminine 'life-giver' (p.29) or simply 'GRACE or LOVE' (p.29). These concepts of a Higher Power sometimes owe much to God images in the psyche as well as to rational reflection. For example, in another study in the USA, one interviewee said: 'I grew up with a very punishing sort of Church of England Protestant [God] . . . I was convinced I was going to hell at the age of eight years old' (Hahn, 2020, p.112). He later came to see his Higher Power as 'a loving parent to his wounded inner child', a transformation that appears to have been effected by working through the 12 steps. Dossett concludes that the language of her interviewees is as much phenomenological as theological, and a rigid separation of religious and secular is not helpful. She finds common features in the discourse of subjects who are 'theists, non-theists and anti-theists' (p.30). Nonetheless, I would argue that this is a theological process of negotiation and interpretation for all. Ordinary and atheological conclusions are often derived in antithesis to certain theological images and concepts, as with one of Dossett's interviewees who reports:

> I don't consider a Higher Power to be a personal being – anthropomorphic – nor an intelligent puppeteer in the sky directing the show. I do not conceive of HP [Higher Power] as a santa god who rewards the good and punishes the naughty. Neither do I see this force as working for some and not others as in 'There but for the Grace of God go I'. (Dossett, 2015, p.29)

Most of my patients with drinking problems, over several decades, were not working 12-step programmes and did not believe in God, but they were able to identify things that mattered deeply to them. Frequently, these were family relationships, often valued more highly after they had been lost through alienating and destructive addictive behaviour. Sometimes they were concerned with self-image, as in the case of one patient who found that he wanted to preserve a 'clean' feeling that he associated with maintaining goals for moderate drinking. Sometimes they were concerned with creative activity, as in the case of a patient who found satisfaction from building model battleships (something that he couldn't do effectively when drinking heavily). These concerns are not explicitly theological, although they might be construed as forms of 'implicit religion' (concerned with commitments, integrating foci and intensive concerns – Bailey, 2010) or spirituality. They are theological, nonetheless, because they bear upon the core concerns of theology with the human condition as manifested in the pathology of addiction. In Buddhism, for example, this relates to craving and attachment (Groves and Farmer, 1994), in Islam to detachment from God (Ali, 2014) and in Christianity to divisions of the will (Cook, 2006).

Other psychiatric disorders are similarly entangled with theology in such a way that the ordinary theologies of patients need to be taken into account in assessment and treatment. I have elsewhere summarised the literature in relation to Christian theological engagements with affective and anxiety disorders, psychosis and various other diagnoses (Cook, 2023b). Much of this arises from constructive theological reflection on lived experience, but some presents obstacles for Christians who might otherwise benefit from engagement with psychiatric services (Huang Harris et al., 2024). Together with my colleagues Isabelle Hamley and John Swinton, I have attempted to address some of the issues that arise for Christians doing their own ordinary theology in the context of mental health challenges (Cook et al., 2023). Elsewhere, members of other faith traditions are engaged in their own theological reflections, for example in Islam (Bagasra, 2023), Hinduism (Kang, 2010) or Buddhism (Nguyen et al., 2012).

Clinical theologies of the future will, I predict, be very different from that envisaged by Frank Lake. They will be much more interdisciplinary in their formal voice and much more phenomenological in their operant voice as they engage with ordinary theological reflections of patients on lived experience. In both cases, whilst they may sometimes be integrative, they will always need to reflect a constructive and critical dialogue between science and religion. This is something that will happen primarily in the clinical consultation, but it also needs to take place within professional discourse, as happens in the Spirituality and Psychiatry Special Interest Group (SPSIG). The clinical role of the psychiatrist is not to defend science in a conflictual way, over and against the ordinary theology of the patient, but rather to act as the skilled therapist assisting the patient to achieve a personal dialogue and/or integration as they reflect on the significance of their illness in relation to their spirituality/faith. In this role, the psychiatrist will need to work collaboratively with mental health chaplains, spiritual care advisers and faith leaders.

There will also, I hope, be much more interfaith dialogue in the future in relation to the shared concerns of people of different religions in the face of the mental health challenges faced by faith communities and wider society. Whilst psychiatry will always be properly patient-centred, the biopsychosocial model reminds us that people are social creatures who flourish best in community, and spirituality/religion are important aspects of that social context. Psychiatry has a contribution to make in support of public mental health (Cook and White, 2018; Long et al., 2024).

Psychiatry and Theology

Psychiatric diagnoses affect human self-understanding in a way that most physical conditions do not. Much of the stigma and prejudice that is faced by people within faith communities has implicit or explicit theological roots, which a critical clinical theology of mental health can effectively challenge. I believe that clinical theology, in the form that I am proposing here, can reinforce positive religious coping, reduce negative religious coping and facilitate positive outcomes in the face of spiritual struggles. Of course, my beliefs and proposals need to be subjected to further empirical research, but meanwhile we cannot ignore the theological elephant in the psychiatric clinic. As part of a whole person, patient-centred approach to mental health care, it is incumbent upon psychiatrists to take into account the spiritual, theological and religious concerns with which their patients struggle.

Spiritual Voices

Spirituality gets entangled with the thinking about psychiatry of both psychiatrists (Chapter 2) and patients (Chapter 3). Even more importantly, at least in terms of its impact upon patients, spirituality gets entangled with psychopathology. The phenomenology of spirituality and the phenomenology of the illness can sometimes be very hard to disentangle. This is not necessarily because the spirituality is pathological, but because – in its very nature – it is concerned with the things that affect us most deeply. When we are ill, our spirituality is therefore expressed in relation to illness. Spirituality (as discussed in the Introduction) cannot be separated conceptually from psychological variables. In relation to mental illness, it is therefore inevitable that the phenomenology of spirituality will become entangled with the phenomenology of the illness – the psychopathology – and with the illness narrative.

Arguably, it is this entanglement which causes the most trouble of all for patients when it comes to the place of spirituality in psychiatry. It makes it difficult for patients to tell their stories of illness without also talking about their spiritual stories. When they do tell these entangled stories, they need to be able to do so without fear of judgement. Sadly, where mental health professionals are concerned, patients often do feel afraid – afraid of being misunderstood and afraid that the things that matter most to them will be deemed pathological or (worse) irrelevant. These entanglements also lead psychiatrists into trouble. It is just so easy to pathologise spirituality (even without meaning to do so) or, worse still, to imagine that one's own spirituality (including atheist or agnostic, as well as religious, spiritualities) can be imposed upon a consultation or a patient.

Spirituality and/or religion influence almost every aspect of mental state, including mood, thought, perception, cognition and insight. Easter celebrations for Christians and hajj pilgrimages for Muslims are emotional experiences. Patients with dementia, even when memory is severely impaired, may remember vividly prayers or music long associated with religious devotion in earlier life. Insight (into illness, adversity and life in general) is crucially coloured by theological interpretations of experience. Untoward events, stresses and painful experiences may be interpreted as punishment from God or demonic attack (both of which are forms of negative religious coping). Centrally, however, it is disorders of thought and perception that become linked to spiritual and religious themes in mental illness, and spiritual and religious experiences are shaped by processes of thinking and perceiving.

Thinking and perceiving are not easily separated. The way in which we experience the world is shaped both by processes of perception and by processes of thinking. It is sometimes pointed out that religious experiences tend to be in keeping with religious and cultural context: 'it is almost always Roman Catholics who have visions of the Virgin and almost always Hindus who have visions of Krishna and extraordinarily rarely, if ever, *vice versa*' (MacIntyre, 1966, p.260). This is indeed true, although some notable exceptions are very interesting. For example, Sundar Singh (1889–c. 1929), born to a Sikh family in North India, was antipathetic towards Christianity and yet had a dramatic conversion experience in which he had a vision of Christ who spoke to him in Hindustani (Cook, 2018, pp.135–136). The story sounds remarkably similar to the conversion of St Paul, as recorded in the Christian New Testament, and yet Singh reported that he did not think that he had previously heard that story at that point in his life.

Given that it is nonetheless usually Christians who see visions (or hear voices) of Christ or Mary, and Hindus who experience visions of Krishna, we may clearly explain this on the basis of cultural conditioning and the 'top down' processes of perception by way of which we tend to see what we expect to see (Cook, 2018, pp.182–183). It is not possible to separate an experience from our interpretation of that experience. The experience is an amalgam of physiological processes of perception and the psychology of predictive processing and interpretation. We may then continue to reflect upon experience, and our interpretations of experience may change, so that it can become very hard to separate exactly what did happen from the evolving stories that we tell about our experience of what happened (Cook, 2018, pp.145–149).

In this chapter, I will focus primarily upon disorders of perception, and especially auditory verbal hallucinations (AVHs), or voice hearing. Readers may well guess that this is because I spent 10 years working as a member of the Wellcome-funded Hearing the Voice project at Durham University, and so it is a topic on which I have reflected a lot over the last decade or two. However, I think that there is also a good argument to be made concerning the importance of voice hearing for our thinking generally about psychiatry and spirituality, both within the world of psychopathology and in the domain of theology and religious studies. It provides a helpful example, or test case, for teasing out some of the broader issues about the phenomenological ways in which spirituality and psychiatry become entangled. Perception and thought, aspects of mental state which are usually distinguished, are also more entangled with each other than is often acknowledged. My colleague Charles Fernyhough (2016), in his book on *The Voices Within*, shows that 'voices' are as much concerned with our own inner dialogue (thoughts) as they are with AVHs. A good place to begin is therefore with a consideration of the nature of voice hearing.

Hearing Voices

Hallucinations are a significant example of the psychopathology for which psychiatrists are on the alert when they conduct a mental state examination. Identification and definition of hallucinations is a key learning objective when training as a psychiatrist. For example, a hallucination may be defined as 'A sensory experience which occurs in the absence of corresponding external stimulation of the relevant sense organ, has a sufficient sense of reality to resemble a veridical perception, over which the subject does not feel s/he has direct and voluntary control, and which occurs in the awake state' (David, 2004, p.110). Auditory verbal hallucinations are thus experiences of this kind – perception-like experiences in the absence of any objectively present stimulus – which occur in the auditory modality and are subjectively heard as voices. However, things are not quite that simple.

When I was a trainee psychiatrist, in the 1980s, I was taught to ask about whether voices were experienced in external space or inner space, and whether they were heard 'out loud' or were more thought-like. The out-loud and external voices were said to be AVHs and the inner thought-like voices were said to be pseudo-hallucinations. According to the thinking of the day, the former had diagnostic significance and the latter did not. This distinction, although still reiterated (e.g., Oyebode, 2023, pp.89, 103–104), now appears to be spurious. Phenomenological research suggests that voices may be recognised on a spectrum from auditory to thought-like, with many having features of both (Woods et al., 2015), and it is not clear that there is a point on that spectrum which discriminates between psychopatho-logical and 'normal' experience.

For most of us, thoughts are inner 'voices', except that we usually recognise them as our own, and we don't hear them out loud. They are not perception-like, except insofar as we might be said to have the capacity to perceive things within our own minds. Thoughts that are not recognised as one's own thoughts may be recognised as a particular kind of thought disorder: thought insertion. However, the phenomenon of thought insertion might also be understood as voices that are not auditory in their perception-like quality. Research on the phenomenology of voice hearing seems to suggest that such voices share a family resemblance with AVHs, rather than thought disorder (Humpston and Broome, 2015).

Recognition of the continuity of thoughts and voices has huge significance, which I do not think psychiatry has yet properly acknowledged. It is a bit like the recognition in physics that energy and matter are interchangeable. Suddenly, you see (or, perhaps better, hear) the world differently. Voice hearing is not about othering people who have alien experiences; it is about the way in which we all listen to, and find meaning in, voices of all kinds. It is, as Fernyhough (2016) has eloquently described, about making sense of the voices within that almost all of us experience in one form or another.

Human thoughts, which for most of us are experienced as internal and largely verbal discourse or dialogue, are a bit like breathing. Most of the time, we breathe unselfcon-sciously and without deliberate effort. Sometimes, we pay close attention to our breathing, perhaps even labouring over it. Similarly, our inner voices are not usually the focus of our conscious attention. We listen to ourselves in an unselfconscious kind of way, and our inner voices naturally and effortlessly help us to focus on, or cause us to be distracted from, other things – our surroundings, other people, our daily routine. When we become more self-conscious about our thinking, what we choose to focus on may be determined by a variety of factors, spiritual or carnal, supernatural or mundane. Thinking can sometimes become hard work and require deliberate effort.

In idle moments, when there is no external distraction, our thoughts – or inner voices – may generate their own distractions. The 'random episodic silent thinking' that takes place at rest seems to be closely related to social cognition (Mars et al., 2012) and is supported by a so-called default mode network of cortical regions of the brain (Mason et al., 2007). Currently, it is not completely clear how the functioning of this network relates to mechan-isms of thought, although we might speculate that stimulus-independent thoughts that form a subjectively important part of our human experience may in some way be related to it (Callard and Margulies, 2014). Taking a more philosophical approach, Daniel Dennett (1991) refers to the 'word-demons' that are part of the 'mental pandemonium' in which a variety of simultaneous mental processes vie for our attention. On this basis, AVHs may simply be the word-demons that shout loudest (Cook, 2018, pp.147–148). As such, they are both our own thoughts and yet not our own thoughts, belonging to the self and yet experienced as in some sense autonomous and alien.

Spiritual/Religious Perceiving

Religion takes a wide variety of forms, some of which (e.g., most forms of Buddhism) are atheistic. Even where religion posits the existence of God, it does not necessarily understand the divine as accessible to human experience, other than in a very general way. In deism, for example, God is understood as non-interventional, revealed in nature and accessible to human reason, but not otherwise humanly accessible, and certainly not by way of the supernatural or miraculous. Some spiritual and religious traditions emphasise a negative, or apophatic, spirituality, whereby it is acknowledged that there will always be much more of God inaccessible to human reason or experience than there is that is accessible using the senses and the rational mind. Nonetheless, for most of the world's major faith traditions, there is also an expectation that God, or the transcendent, is accessible to human experience, however imperfectly or provisionally.

This accessibility to human experience may be mediated in various ways – including mystical experiences, circumstances perceived as providential, religious rituals, acts of charity and a variety of perceptual phenomena, some of which might fulfil the technical definition of hallucinations, albeit they are not interpreted as such in a religious context. Some such experiences are mundane and ordinary. As St Teresa of Avila famously wrote, 'the Lord walks among the pots and pans' in the kitchen (Kavanaugh and Rodriguez, 1985, pp.119–120). Amongst these diverse experiences, the hearing of voices is a significant contributor to the fabric of what we call religion. Drawing on the work of Ann Taves (2011), I have suggested elsewhere that voices may be understood as one of the 'building blocks' of religion (Cook, 2018, pp.39, 226, 2022d, pp.315–316). They stand at an important intersection of the transcendent and the immanent, the imaginable and the ineffable, of mystery and reason.

Scripture, in most of the world's faith traditions, plays a part in affirming this key, mediatory role of voices. In Islam, for example, the Qur'an is traditionally understood as having been revealed to Mohammed by the angel Gabriel. The Qur'an (Surah 4:163–164) itself affirms the prophetic experience as one of inspiration by God, or as a kind of divine 'speech':

> We have sent thee
> Inspiration, as We sent it
> To Noah and the Messengers
> After him: We sent
> Inspiration to Abraham,
> Ishmael, Isaac, Jacob
> And the Tribes, to Jesus,
> Job, Jonah, Aaron, and Solomon,
> And to David We gave
> The Psalms.
>
> Of some Messengers We have
> Already told thee the story;
> Of others we have not –
> And to Moses Allah spoke direct –

(Ali, 2000)

God's speech is not, however, usually so 'direct' and most Muslims (similarly Christians and Jews) would not presume to have heard God in the same way that Moses did. Nonetheless, the principle is established in the three major monotheistic traditions that God may in some sense 'speak', whether directly or via an intermediary such as an angel, and that the voice of God may thus – one way or another – be 'heard'. A similar case may be made for the importance of voices in other faith traditions, including Zoroastrianism, Mormonism, Bahaism and Hinduism (Cook, 2018, pp.51–55). These inner voices might be referred to according to a diverse vocabulary. In the Quaker tradition, a visual metaphor is primarily employed, that of the inner, or inward, light (Cook, 2018, pp.132–133). In so-called New Age spirituality, there is reference to 'channelling' (Spencer, 2010). Sometimes, the voices may be referred to as thoughts – as in the expression that 'God put a thought into my mind' (Dein and Cook, 2015). In very broad terms, they may be referred to simply as 'inspirations'. For Jenny, in Chapter 1, they were a kind of prompting. Sometimes, and probably most frequently, they are referred to as voices.

In some strands of Christianity, this literal experience of hearing a voice is both normative and encouraged, as exemplified in the research findings of Tanya Luhrmann (2012) in her studies of the Vineyard churches of California and Chicago. In some religions, such as spiritualism, the voices of spiritual entities may be perceived by certain people (mediums) understood as particularly gifted (Powell and Moseley, 2021). For others, including many Christians, the divine voice might be understood not so much as literal as metaphorical, not so much a matter of perception, more as one of discernment and interpretation. Voices which might be described as spiritual in some way, perhaps as the speech of immaterial spirits, demons or angels rather than as theologically 'divine', are also recognised by some who would identify themselves as spiritual but not religious (SBNR) rather than traditionally 'religious'. Indeed, one way or another, the principle that voices may emerge from a spiritual domain and, as such, should be carefully listened to is enshrined in scripture and/or tradition, in belief and in human experience, for many (and probably the vast majority of) people worldwide. Even if most people do not experience the hearing of voices (i.e., voices not identified as their own thoughts) on a daily basis, or even infrequently, the idea of the possibility of hearing spiritual voices is there in the collective psyche.

In one way or another, this worldwide ubiquity of beliefs about spiritual voices creates expectations which influence both the nature and the interpretation of spiritual and religious experience. Because these beliefs are widely embedded in culture and society, they do not necessarily confine themselves to religious people. In one comparative study of religious and non-religious voice hearers, in the non-religious group of patients with psychosis, 23 per cent attributed a religious identity to the voice(s) that they heard (Cottam et al., 2011).

In one memorable encounter, many years ago, an atheist colleague sought out my advice concerning experiences which she had found unsettling. These experiences turned out to be hypnopompic hallucinations of a golden figure whom she identified as Christ. Not being a religious person, she found these experiences unwanted and confusing. 'I do not want to become a Christian!', she told me. In this case, there were no voices, only visions. However, her experience of the disjunction between personal belief and perception-like experience was one which she found difficult to accept and I learnt a lot from her as we discussed the cognitive dissonance that arose from it. I was able to reassure her, as a psychiatrist, that her experiences were not a sign of mental illness. As a fellow human being, I was only able to accompany her on the beginning of a process of finding meaning in them. This certainly did not entail any kind of proselytising, which would have been an abuse of my professional role, but it did involve a person-centred approach to spiritual experience within which I was able to affirm her search for meaning. The important part of the conversation was not so much the elucidation of phenomenology (although that was important) as the discernment of meaning within the experience.

Spiritual voices may thus, for the clinician, offer important clinical information in support of particular diagnoses. For the patient, they may be a source of distress, a symptom which they would (usually) like not to have. However, within a spiritual or religious context, they may also be deeply meaningful. As such, the clinical or pastoral task is not so much to make a diagnosis or relieve distress (although both of these things may also be very important) as to facilitate the search for meaning.

Spiritually Significant Voices

The hearing of voices has historically been associated with mental illness and it is only over the last three decades or so that it has become clear that the experience is common in the general population in the absence of diagnosed mental disorder (Cook, 2018, p.7). It is also common as an element of spiritual or religious experience, albeit often not referred to as 'voice hearing' in this context. There are thus different contexts in which voices are heard: the world of psychiatry and mental health, the wider world of voice hearing (e.g., the Hearing Voices Network) and the world of spiritual and religious experience. There are phenomenological continuities and discontinuities between the experiences of voices in these different contexts, but it is not a priori clear that these experiences are fundamentally different in themselves. The continuities, the core family resemblance of voice hearing experiences, present a number of problems for psychiatry and for theology and spirituality.

If I hear a voice which, as I understand it, is God telling me to serve the poor in India, is this evidence of mental illness or might it – just possibly – be God? The historically atheistic presuppositions of psychiatry do not help here as they have often prejudiced psychiatrists against widely held – and in many cases culturally normative – beliefs that God does in fact speak to people (however frequently or rarely that might be expected in different traditions). Such experiences are also problematic for spirituality, religion and theology. Even if I accept that God does sometimes speak to people (whatever that might mean), it is also clear that people sometimes believe God is speaking to them when others, including members of the same faith community, might widely assert that God is not. Examples of such disagreements range from the trivial and mundane through to matters of life and death.

By way of clarifying the 'life and death' end of this spectrum, two examples may be offered here. Joan of Arc, later canonised by the Catholic Church, turned the course of the Hundred Years War in Europe because she was obedient to her voices and because the message that they conveyed was seen by her and by others as politically inspirational. She was burnt as a heretic because her voices were deemed, by a politically biased ecclesiastical court convened by her enemies, not to have been from God (Cook, 2023a, pp.71–86). In this case, the voices heard by one woman significantly altered the course of history. In other cases, it is the voices of a religious movement that impact upon the lives of individuals. In the wave of religious enthusiasm that swept across the continent during the European Reformation, the authority of the Catholic Church was challenged not only by the rational theological arguments of figures such as Luther and Calvin but also by others claiming direct inspiration from God. In fact, these enthusiasts often challenged both Protestant and Catholic norms by way of apocalyptic expectations and their unconventional and sometimes patently immoral behaviour. In one notorious case, a young man decapitated his brother, claiming that this was the command of God. He was then himself sentenced to death (Heyd, 1995, pp.15–18).

It is not only the voices claimed to be from God that cause trouble. People also hear evil voices, such as those of Satan or of demons. These experiences may lead to even more complex theological questions as to the nature of evil, which are not soluble by psychiatric phenomenology operating on its own but rather require an interdisciplinary response. The voices described in the contemporary account of one patient provide a good example (Barber, 2016). When these voices were first experienced, they were interpreted by clergy from whom she initially sought help as evidence of demon possession, and subsequently by mental health professionals as evidence of illness. It was some years before she found a place within which spiritual and psychiatric perspectives could be integrated. Psychiatry is an inherently interdisciplinary endeavour, drawing on the full range of neurosciences and social sciences, but it is much more selective in its engagement with the humanities, and very wary of any engagement with theology. Sadly, the sentiments are reciprocated by many clergy and faith leaders who remain wary of engaging with the insights of psychiatry.

Voices may have spiritual/religious significance either because the identity of the voice is experienced as spiritual/religious (e.g., God, angels, demons, etc.) or because the voice has a message of spiritual significance (e.g., calling to a vocation as a priest, or accusing the hearer of sin/guilt). The discernment of this meaning, and its negotiation with others in a family or faith community, is a theological enterprise, not a psychiatric one. However, it raises some significant questions about whether, and how, the psychiatric process of discernment (leading to diagnosis) interacts with the theological process of discerning spiritual meaning. Writing about a curious and tragic train of events in seventeenth-century France, in which a whole community became embroiled in controversy surrounding supposed demonic intervention in the lives of a group of Ursuline nuns, Aldous Huxley observed: 'by no means all inspirations are divine, or even moral, even relevant. How are we to distinguish between the leadings of a not-I who is the Holy Spirit and of that other not-I who is sometimes an imbecile, sometimes a lunatic, and sometimes a malevolent criminal?' (Huxley, 1971, pp.89–90). This all-important question of how we are to discern the meaning, source and trustworthiness of voices involves multiple elements, not least that of spiritual discernment, to which we will return later. At this juncture, however, it raises questions as to whether one can make a differential diagnosis between experiences of the Holy Spirit (to use Huxley's vocabulary) and those of mental illness (to use a contemporary term in preference to Huxley's vocabulary).

Differential Diagnosis

A common approach to dealing with the entanglement of psychopathology with spiritual/religious experience is to suggest that a differential diagnosis needs to be made between 'true', or genuine, spiritual/religious experience and psychopathology indicative of mental illness. A variety of criteria have been suggested by way of which the distinction can be judged. For example, Andrew Sims (2016, pp.25–38) suggested that the distinction may be made on the basis of criteria for distinguishing psychopathology from normal mental phenomena, knowledge of the spiritual/religious context, the life narrative and common sense. This may be very helpful in many cases, but sadly common sense is often in short supply, and is sometimes compromised by stigma and prejudice.

De Menezes and Moreira-Almeida (2009) offer a longer and more specific list of criteria by way of which the proposed distinction may be made. Thus, genuine spiritual experience, as distinguished from psychopathology, is said to be characterised by: lack of psychological suffering; absence of social and occupational impairments; short duration of the experience; critical attitude (to have doubts about the reality of the experience); compatibility with the patient's cultural or religious group; no co-morbidities; control over the experience; personal growth over time; and experience directed towards helping others. These criteria are certainly all helpful in a general way of understanding someone's experience. However, they are also quite debatable in terms of their discriminative validity. Lack of psychological suffering, absence of impairments and control over the experience, for example, would place many mystics within mainstream faith traditions on the wrong side of the boundary between spiritual experience and mental disorder. Compatibility with cultural/religious group would also depend upon the group, or part of a group, with which one identifies. St John of the Cross and St Teresa of Avila were notably identified as deviant by some members of their religious order within late medieval Catholic Spain but held up as exemplary by others.

In a recent systematic review, Mosqueiro et al. (2023) argued that negative symptoms, functional impairments and cognitive/behavioural disorganisation are better guides to differential diagnosis between pathological and non-pathological 'anomalous experiences' than is the actual phenomenology of these (perception-like) experiences in themselves. Such a consideration is undoubtedly helpful in undertaking a psychiatric differential diagnosis. However, it is not necessarily helpful in making a spiritual assessment, or in interpreting the spiritual meaning and significance of the experiences concerned in their whole life context (of which a diagnosis is just one part).

Significant concerns about all such criteria arise on both theological and scientific grounds. Is it legitimate or meaningful to understand a binary, and mutually exclusive, distinction between 'normal' and pathological spiritual experience? Why might someone not be having a theologically meaningful spiritual experience in the context of a diagnosable mental disorder? Some spiritually significant voices occur in times of crisis, and one might expect that – if spirituality or faith is meaningful as a coping resource – such experiences might sometimes accompany the distress and disorientation of mental illness and be experienced as positive coping resources at such times. Empirical research seems to support this approach. Thus, Arjan Braam, Eva Ouwehand and their colleagues in the Netherlands (Ouwehand et al., 2018) have shown that spiritual experiences accompanying acute episodes of bipolar disorder are identified by patients as spiritually meaningful even after their recovery from the episode of illness. It is possible, at least according to the testimony of those concerned, to have experiences of illness which are associated both with psychopathology and with spiritual meaning.

'Genuine' spiritual experiences, or perhaps it's better to say 'spiritually significant' experiences, and psychopathology are thus not mutually exclusive. They are completely different kinds of things. Whereas psychopathology is diagnostically significant, leading to confirmation or exclusion of particular diagnoses as present or absent (as defined within taxonomies such as International Classification of Diseases (ICD) or Diagnostic and Statistical Manual of Mental Disorders (DSM)), the phenomenology of spiritual experience is interpreted according to a completely different framework of suppositions. Spiritual experience is not a binary state, either present or absent, genuine or false; it is open to interpretation in an almost infinite variety of ways. It is never 'absent', albeit the right of some people not to describe their experiences as spiritual must be respected. It is amenable, for those who are so inclined, to various interpretations which may be more or less meaningful, more or less valid, depending upon the criteria for discernment which are brought to bear upon them.

The making of a differential diagnosis between psychopathology and 'genuine' spiritual phenomena risks epistemic injustice – a failure to take seriously the testimony and interpretations of the patient regarding their own spiritual experiences. All patients are having spiritual experiences which need to be seen as genuine, in their own way, and treated with respect, even if they are in various ways entangled with psychopathology. This concern will be discussed further in the next section of this chapter ('Epistemic Injustice'). The important consideration here is that the genuineness, or spiritual significance, of experiences is not entirely dependent upon psychiatric diagnosis or upon the phenomenology that helps in making such a diagnosis. Differential diagnosis (of the psychopathology vs 'genuine' spiritual experience kind) easily implies that the spiritual experiences of psychiatric patients should not be taken seriously, that they are somehow less spiritual people or that psychopathology cannot be the basis of a 'genuine' spiritual experience. The imposition of the process of differential diagnosis in this way perpetuates a form of stigma that attaches itself to mental disorder and is thus something which psychiatrists and other mental health professionals should strive to combat, not reinforce.

The making of differential diagnoses between psychopathology and spiritual phenomena prioritises the role of the psychiatrist as the one who determines whether or not experiences are spiritually 'genuine' or meaningful (by a process of exclusion), whereas such a role is usually much better facilitated by others (as a positive process), including clergy, chaplains or spiritual directors. The danger is that the psychiatrist becomes the arbiter of what counts, spiritually speaking, rather than affirming the spirituality of all patients and working collaboratively with colleagues in spiritual care.

The approach proposed here is thus one of not making a differential diagnosis but, rather, conducting independent and parallel assessments of psychopathology and spiritual phenomena, both of which need to be evaluated and interpreted on their own terms. The presence of psychopathology, psychiatric interpretation of which implies a particular psychiatric diagnosis, does not imply that spiritual experiences are 'false' or meaningless. The absence of a psychiatric diagnosis does not necessarily mean that reported spiritual experiences are 'genuine' or that they should necessarily be interpreted spiritually as meaning what someone says they mean. Psychiatric assessment and spiritual discernment are entangled and interrelated in complex ways which are not amenable to simple binary distinctions. Neither are they 'non-overlapping magisteria' (as discussed in Chapter 4). Spiritual context and interpretation are matters to be taken into account by psychiatrists in assessing phenomenology, and differential diagnosis is essential in psychiatric assessment of psychopathology, for the purpose of determining diagnosis. Psychiatric diagnosis is a factor to be taken into account, alongside others, in processes of spiritual discernment. However, differential diagnosis is not helpful as a tool to discriminate between 'genuine' and psychopathological spiritual experiences; indeed, the whole idea of 'genuine', in this context, is very unhelpful. There may or may not be a diagnosis, but there is always (for those who wish to seek it out) spiritual meaning to be found in life's experiences, however anomalous or unusual they might be.

Epistemic Injustice

When it comes to those whose spiritually significant voices are associated with a diagnosis of a mental disorder, there is a significant problem of epistemic injustice (Cullinan et al., 2024). This not only is a problem in relation to spirituality but represents a broader issue in psychiatry, whereby those identified as patients are not taken seriously as knowing agents. This problem is not helped by referring to 'service users' or 'experts by experience' instead of using the traditional term 'patient'. Indeed, in some ways, these changes of vocabulary make things worse, implying that it is only as a consumer of services (rather than as a fellow human being) that someone has to be shown respect, or that simply having an experience makes one an expert (which it does not). This problem is not one that only concerns psychiatry. Within faith communities, and within a wider world of non-religious spirituality, there is a complex search for meaning in which some are not taken seriously merely by virtue of having received a diagnosis of a mental disorder. This does not happen in quite the same way in the wider world of medicine. If you are dying of cancer and hear a comforting voice in which you find spiritual and theological meaning, you are likely to be taken seriously (at least by members of your faith community, but hopefully also medical professionals and others). If you are suffering from schizophrenia and have a similar experience, it is likely that you will be told that this is a symptom of your illness.

None of this should be taken to imply that clinicians, chaplains, faith leaders or others have to agree with the interpretation of experience offered by every patient in regard to every experience. As a clergy colleague used to tell me, in relation to the kinds of experiences discussed in Chapter 6, 'experience is sacred; interpretation is free'. I listen to my patients with respect for the sacredness of their experience, but I am free to interpret these experiences in my own way, according to my psychiatric and/or theological training. Indeed, it is essential to the overcoming of epistemic injustice that patients are not patronised by blanket agreement with whatever they may say about the spiritual/religious significance of their experiences. At the same time, it is important that the significance of their experiences is not dismissed out of hand. Interpretation of such experiences requires a careful process of spiritual and theological discernment.

These problems are only a part of the wider entanglement of spirituality and psychiatry, within which prejudice and discrimination operate in a variety of ways to the detriment of patients and/or those who identify as having a particular spiritual or theological perspective at the same time as they experience mental illness. They are not adequately addressed by re-emphasising the boundaries between the world of spirituality, faith and theology over and against the world of psychiatry. Rather, they require interdisciplinary and multidisciplinary engagement, mutual understanding and collaboration between mental health professionals, chaplaincy/spiritual care and faith communities. They also require a fundamental change within psychiatry towards the recognition that human beings seek meaning – including spiritual meaning – in their lives. To tell people that their experiences are not meaningful, because they are a feature of an illness, does not promote human flourishing but rather degrades it. A core aim of psychiatry, within its remit to adopt a person-centred and holistic approach to illness, should be facilitation and encouragement of the search for meaning. Of course, this does not mean that we have to agree with particular interpretations of meaning, which is a matter for spiritual discernment, but only with the general principle that experiences are meaningful.

Presence, Social Agency and Affective Valence

A key finding of recent research on voice hearing is that a voice is never just a voice. In our work in the Hearing the Voice project in Durham, we met with a variety of voice hearers from different perspectives. One such participant reported the experience that 'The voices are here now, but they are not speaking'. Many voice hearers report that their voices are accompanied by a sense of presence (Cheyne, 2012; Alderson-Day, 2023). Voices are also commonly reported as being characterful (Woods et al., 2015). They have personality and speak in different tones of voice, conveying calm or anger, kindness or hostility, and being affirming or derogatory. One voice hearer referred to her voice as her 'best friend', whereas for another the voices were demonic. Voice hearing is thus rarely only about a voice. It is about social relationship with an experienced 'other'.

Voices – as experienced by those who hear them – thus have an identity. This may be of spiritual/religious or autobiographical significance. Positively, this voice may be the voice of God, or of spirits, saints or angels. As such it is often found to be comforting, encouraging, affirming and positively meaningful. For others, voices are identified as demons or malign spirits of some kind and are correspondingly evil or abusive, demeaning, critical and negatively meaningful.

Voices, having social agency, may be conversation partners or may issue commands. Contrary to traditional psychiatric thinking, command hallucinations do not necessarily have diagnostic significance, but they may have spiritual significance. Conversation with voices may be a positive experience or unpleasant (especially if the voices are identified as evil). Where they are identified as divine, their instructions may be taken seriously but are not necessarily obeyed. One research participant in Tanya Luhrmann's landmark study in the Vineyard churches in California and Chicago believed that God had told her to start a school – but she never did (Luhrmann, 2012, p.233). For others, including participants in our own research (Cook et al., 2022), a voice gave instructions at a key turning point in their lives, leading to their religious conversion, or to fulfilling vocations such as teaching or priesthood.

Perhaps the single most psychiatrically significant feature of voices is that they have affective valence (De Leede-Smith and Barkus, 2013). Hearing the voice of God, or a voice that you identify as a friend or an angel, tends to be associated with peace or, even if somewhat frightening, is still perceived as a life-enriching and encouraging experience. Hearing the voices of demons or evil spirits (or of a past abuser) tends to be associated with fear and anxiety in such a way as to be life-denying, denigrating and discouraging. Those whose voices have negative affective valence tend to seek help – including psychiatric help – whereas those with positive affective valence do not.

Quantifying Voices

Qualitative aspects of voice hearing, such as affective valence or the experienced identity of the voice, have considerable importance for the voice hearer in terms of the nature and meaning of the experience. However, quantitative aspects of the experience are also important. Those who hear voices are usually able to say how often they hear them, how many voices they identify and how long they have been experiencing them. There are no hard and fast rules here but – as something of an overgeneralisation – spiritually significant voices seem to be fewer in number (often only one) and less frequent, in comparison with other kinds of voice hearing (Cook et al., 2022). There are, however, within this grouping those who have ongoing, sometimes daily, conversations with their voice, especially in cases where the voice is identified as the voice of God.

The number and identity of voices is influenced by religious tradition. For Muslims, the voice of God might be heard, albeit (according to the limited data available, e.g., Suhail and Cochrane, 2002) not by most. For Christians, some distinguish between the voice of God (the Father), the voice of Jesus and the voice of the Holy Spirit (Cook et al., 2022). There are also voices of saints, angels and demons to be heard in Christianity and in other traditions, giving rise to a rich variety of identifiable sources which might potentially be spiritually significant.

Once-in-a-lifetime spiritually significant voices seem to have particular importance in terms of identity, vocation and belief, and are sometimes associated with far-reaching and life-transforming consequences (Cook et al., 2022). They usually have positive affective valence. They may be associated with conversion; one of our research subjects heard a voice that said, 'Be baptised', in this context. For others they are associated with a vocational calling, such as one of our subjects who heard a voice that said, 'Teach scripture!', and went on to become a religious education teacher. On the other hand, they may be associated with a life crisis, the need for comfort amidst adversity ('Do not be afraid!') or the need for confirmation/clarification of the way forward amidst difficult life circumstances. One woman, on meeting her future husband, heard a voice that said, 'You're going to marry him, you know!'.

Spiritually significant voices that occur more frequently, and sometimes daily, may be quite conversational and/or associated with a sense of companionable presence (Cook et al., 2022). They may be experienced in the context of prayer. For some Christians, and others, relationship with God is experienced in terms of ongoing conversation, often about mundane matters. An interesting historical example of this kind is found in Margery Kempe, a fourteenth-century English woman whose autobiography records ongoing, daily conversations with God, Jesus, the virgin Mary, saints and angels (Cook, 2023a, pp.21–41). Examples of this kind are also recorded by Tanya Luhrmann in her research in charismatic Christian churches in the USA.

The 'once in a lifetime' and 'conversational' categories are ideal types. It is clear that there are complex cases that fall somewhere in between the two, in terms of frequency and qualitative significance, and that other experiences of spiritually significant voice hearing are not easily categorised or quantified.

Context and Significance

The voices that I have called 'spiritually significant', which are usually not associated with a psychiatric diagnosis (Cook et al., 2022), gain their spiritual/religious significance in relation to context and circumstances. As in some of the earlier examples, this may be religious conversion, life crises or practices of spiritual devotion and prayer. For those that do occur in the context of a psychiatric disorder, the nature of that diagnosis and its concomitant psychopathology also need to be taken into account in discerning meaning and planning spiritual/clinical care. However, in the research undertaken by Ouwehand et al. (2018), a psychiatric diagnosis does not necessarily negate meaning, biographical or theological significance, or the personal value placed upon experiences arising in the course of illness.

In our study of spiritually significant voices (Cook et al., 2022), which were primarily not associated with a psychiatric diagnosis, participants reported that their voice-hearing experiences were 'life-enhancing', 'wonderful', 'precious' and strengthening. These were clearly – for the majority – experiences which facilitated coping, and brought a sense of connection, gratitude, confidence, spiritual growth and acceptance.

Voices in Psychosis

Voices heard in the context of a psychotic illness are often not positive experiences: 'While sometimes a source of comfort or companionship, voices in psychotic disorders are more often unsettling, undermining, or abusive, and cause significant suffering and disturbance within people's lives' (Woods et al., 2022, p.6). The extent to which such voices are identified as spiritual/religious in some way is variously defined, and varies significantly over time and across geographical locations (Cook, 2015). However, it does seem that the spiritual/religious message of these voices still relates to context and is meaningful.

Furthermore, the exploration of voices in an interview is a collaborative venture. Reflecting on a series of research interviews with people hearing voices in psychosis, Tehseen Noorani suggests that there is a complex and constant renegotiating of the process of data gathering: 'This analysis troubles several common assumptions about the interview format: that it transparently represents what knowers know, that knowledge about self is straightforwardly accessible, and that the continuity of experience is recalled, rather than worked out together' (Noorani, 2022, p.107). I would suggest that this process of negotiating and renegotiating also takes place in clinical interviews and that clinicians therefore need to take great care to remember that they are 'working out together' with patients what can be known about their voices and that this knowledge is not 'straightforwardly accessible'. In relation to religion and spirituality, for example, Noorani notes that interviewees tended to respond only in relation to religion, and thus negatively, but that there were numerous spiritual themes within the interviews (pp.105–106).

Voices often arise in the context of a history of trauma and so the conversation about the voices easily becomes a locus of the search for meaning in the wake of deeply painful life experiences which challenge settled and comfortable worldviews, including those offered by spirituality or religion. Reflecting on a research interview, in the same volume as Noorani, I suggested that the voices of a woman called Leah, in this case explicitly spiritual in nature, reflected struggles taking place in both her inner and her outer worlds (Cook, 2022b). They were at the same time distressing and a means of coping with that distress. Given that positive spiritual/religious coping offers an important social and psychological resource for dealing with adversity, it is important in clinical practice to be able to engage with patients in a collaborative process of making sense of such experiences and then exploring ways in which spirituality/religion may be seen as a component of treatment, rather than merely a dimension of the psychopathology.

In her studies of patients with bipolar disorder, Eva Ouwehand (2020, pp.47–72) found that spiritual/religious experiences were less common (or rather were manifested as an absence/poverty of spiritual experience) in acute episodes of depression as contrasted with acute episodes of mania. In the latter, voices contributed to perceptions of transcendental/divine reality and sense of mission/vocation. Negatively valued experiences during mania (e.g., fear) were mostly devoid of religious content. Patients reported a 'sliding scale' of continuity of spiritual/religious experiences between periods when they were euthymic and manic (although, unfortunately, specific data are not provided in relation to voices/hallucinations).

What Ouwehand refers to as a 'sliding scale', others may nuance differently and, in some cases, it is clear that there is marked discontinuity between spiritual experiences in and out of acute psychosis. This does not necessarily mean that they cannot be positively transformational. Isabel Clarke et al. (2016), for example, have developed a concept of 'high schizotypy' (not to be confused with schizotypal personality disorder) within which they envisage that people have 'ease of access to "non-ordinary experiencing"' which might include 'previously excluded spiritual perspectives' (p.114). For Clarke and colleagues, the important tasks of the clinician are to respect the experience and to 'retain an open mind about the possibility of connection and influence beyond the self for those in a state of openness' (p.118). They suggest that, in talking with patients, it is helpful to distinguish between shared and unshared reality as a way of maintaining a therapeutic alliance and managing 'the twin dangers of collusion and invalidation' (p.118).

In employing terms such as 'high schizotypy' (or similar categories designated by different names, such as 'transliminality' – see Thalbourne and Delin, 1994), Clarke and others go further than I would wish to do in blurring the boundaries between psychosis and wider mystical/spiritual experience. Whilst it may well be the case that some mystics in the world's major spiritual/religious traditions were psychotic, this would not seem to me to be the norm. Nor do all of the states that Clarke et al. explore include the hearing of voices. In only one of the three cases that they discusses in their chapter on 'Narratives of transformation in psychosis' are voices a prominent feature. However, voices do appear as a prominent feature in many of the mystical experiences of the world's major faith traditions and the question does therefore arise as to how the relationship between the voices of psychosis and mystical experience might best be understood.

My own proposal is that the continuities and discontinuities between different kinds of voice hearing (e.g., spiritually significant voices and the voices of psychosis) need to be acknowledged. Whilst they have a certain phenomenological family resemblance, they also have differences (at least in degree, if not also in qualitative kind). More importantly, the extent to which they are found meaningful in (what Clarke et al. might call) shared reality is a matter for sociocultural and spiritual discernment that goes beyond the bounds of normally accepted psychiatric practice. One of the dangers of over-emphasising the similarities, particularly in the practice of psychiatry, is that it further reinforces the stereotype of the psychiatrist as areligious and reductionistic, reducing the categories of spiritual and religious tradition to those of psychiatry.

Amir

I was asked to see Amir by a clinical psychologist working with a psychosis team. During the time that I saw him he seemed to be generally well maintained on antipsychotic medication, prescribed for a schizoaffective disorder. However, he continued to be preoccupied with a variety of spiritual concerns, which he did not feel that the team adequately understood. Furthermore, he felt that his medication 'blunted' his spiritual awareness and was keen that the dosage should be reduced as soon as possible. There was the constant concern amongst the multidisciplinary team that he would stop taking his medication.

At the heart of Amir's distress was a concern that he should be telling people about the apocalyptic visions that he was having, which he believed were premonitions, in order to avert a global disaster. He had repeatedly been to the police station to tell them about these visions, and they had told him that they didn't want to hear from him about this anymore.

He was feeling guilty that he had a gift and a responsibility to use it for the good of humankind, but that he was not warning people of what was going to happen.

At the same time, Amir was engaged in a range of personal spiritual practices drawing on the traditions of Christianity, Buddhism and Spiritism. Mostly, these did not take the form of supplicatory prayer, nor were they directed explicitly towards God, but rather involved meditative practices within which he 'encountered' various spiritual figures, including the archangel Michael and a spirit guide whom he called Oshango. He held conversations with these spirit beings whose voices might be considered merely imaginary or perhaps (according to traditional categories) pseudo-hallucinations. However, to Amir, they were very real and not products of his own imagination. He considered that his ability to hear the voices of these beings was a gift of clairaudience.[1]

Amir was not a regular member of any church or other religious group and his syncretistic spirituality took a very individualistic emphasis. He had discussed his experiences with various spiritual mentors, including a Buddhist monk. He was also receptive to discussing these experiences with me and appreciated my affirmation of the importance of his spiritual life, but had very strongly held beliefs which were not generally open to negotiation with others. During the course of our conversations, I was amused to discover that I had given similar advice to the Buddhist monk, particularly in terms of encouraging him to simplify the range and diversity of his spiritual practices (which were occupying a considerable amount of his time each day), but that he had not felt inclined to heed the advice given by either of us.

It might well be argued that my intervention in this case added little to what my chaplaincy colleagues (and the Buddhist monk) were already offering in terms of spiritual support. However, the 'bridge' between the medical and the spiritual was important to Amir and – I believe – reinforced his otherwise equivocal willingness to engage with medical treatment. I was also able to advise the clinical team that most of Amir's beliefs, practices and experiences were within what might be considered the 'normal range' of various spiritual/religious traditions and were not, in themselves, delusional. Of course, his intense preoccupation with these matters, and the amount of time that they were taking in his life, were a concern and may well have been exacerbated by his illness. Careful attention to matters of epistemic justice, and affirmation of the importance of Amir's spiritual life, provided a more constructive and collaborative approach to treatment than the labelling of spiritual phenomena as psychopathology. More importantly, they affirmed Amir as a person for whom we (as a clinical team) had empathy and respect.

Amir's apocalyptic preoccupations seemed much more directly a product of his illness. In other circumstances, it would have been good to talk with a member of his church or congregation to establish the extent to which his beliefs were shared with others in the same faith community. However, Amir was a bit of a loner and not a regular member of any local religious group. To the extent that he had discussed things with the Buddhist monk, it seemed as though my concerns about his spiritual preoccupations were shared by others. The form, if not also the content, of his apocalyptic beliefs seemed clearly delusional. If I had wanted to make a differential diagnosis, I would have seen this as evidence of psychosis rather than 'normal' spirituality. However, it was not clear to me that this was a helpful distinction to make; rather, the promotion of positive spiritual coping was a more beneficial

---

[1] A term borrowed from spiritualist and paranormal literature relating to the gift of hearing voices from the spiritual realm.

intervention than a fruitless discussion about the details of Amir's apocalypticism. Of course, none of this precluded the possibility of also adjusting Amir's dosage of medication, but he continued to be resistant to this because of his perception that it adversely affected his spiritual awareness.

Spiritual Voices

For most (non-deistic) theistic spiritualities, whether religious or not, the question inevitably arises as to how a personal transcendent reality is understood to relate to the immanent order of human life, and especially a broadly conceived domain of object relations, including spiritual as well as human others. Theology has a variety of possible solutions to this question, not least those instantiated in apophatic spiritualities which emphasise not-knowing, rather than knowing, in relationship to God. However, most spiritual and religious traditions also have their cataphatic theologies, emphasising what can be known, and most people who identify as spiritual and/or religious seek to listen to the inner (and outer) voices that might be a means of (for want of a better phrase) 'hearing the voice of God'. This affirmation of the importance of spiritual listening may take many forms, but the hearing of spiritual voices (whether understood metaphorically, subjectively or literally) is one of the most common, worldwide.

The 'spiritually significant voices' that I have identified in this chapter are generally concerned with the non-pathological phenomenology of this spiritual listening. The empirical research that I have cited focusses on predominantly Judeo-Christian research samples, but literature from the study of religion would suggest that the phenomenon (in its many and varied forms) is much wider than this. In the context of mental illness, unsurprisingly, psychopathology becomes entangled with spirituality and religion in disorders of thought and perception. It is the task of the good psychiatrist not to try to disentangle these so much as to discern wisely which threads of thought and perception belong more to one than to the other, and to lead the patient to a place of being able to make creative sense of the tangle (as much as is possible) in a meaningful, integrative and life-affirming way.

Demon Possession

Chapter

6

If spirituality and religion are concerned with things that matter most deeply to people, then they can present a source of deep distress when they go wrong, or when they are associated with psychological struggles or threats. Spiritual struggles may be defined as 'experiences of tension, conflict or strain that centre on whatever people view as sacred' (Pargament and Exline, 2022, p.6). Such struggles are not uncommon. Although the term 'spiritual struggles' is used more or less interchangeably with 'negative religious coping', the two are not exactly the same. Spiritual struggles do not necessarily always have negative outcomes. They also have the potential to bring about spiritual and/or psychological growth (Pargament and Exline, 2022, pp.8–9).

Amongst the various kinds of spiritual struggles that people may face, demonic struggles are concerned with experiences interpreted as owing to a maleficent, supernatural enemy. They are thus believed to be encounters with personal evil, with demons, hostile spirits, the Devil or other non-benevolent spiritual entities. Such beliefs are not necessarily delusional, given that most of the world's faith traditions have some conception of evil forces in opposition to the divine. Nor are such beliefs unusual in the Western world. In the 2005 Baylor Religion survey in the USA, 75 per cent of respondents reported that they 'absolutely' or 'probably' believed in the existence of Satan and 70 per cent in the existence of demons. In a study of 343 mainly Protestant outpatients in Switzerland, 38 per cent believed that their problems may have been caused by evil spirits (Pfeifer, 1994, 1999). In one study of Protestant Christians in Australia (Hartog and Gow, 2005), 38 per cent expressed a belief that demons could cause depression, and 37 per cent that they could cause schizophrenia.

Belief in demons can have negative effects on mental health (Nie and Olson, 2016). Experiences of demonic struggles may well be frightening and distressing (e.g., Abu-Raiya et al., 2015a, 2015b) and may even have an impact on mortality (Pargament et al., 2001). When demonic struggles become entangled with psychopathology, they are likely to represent complex diagnostic and therapeutic challenges.

It is in the nature of such experiences that they are at an interface between religion and psychiatry, and that they are contested and controversial. Psychiatry has historically been closely involved with trying to understand how they arise and how they should be treated. A whole chapter was devoted to demonomania in Jean-Étienne Esquirol's *Mental Maladies*, published originally in French in 1838 (Esquirol, 1845). Freud published a case study of what he called a 'demonological neurosis' in 1922 (Freud, 1985b, pp. 377–423). For Jung, possession provided keys to understanding the relationship between a conscious ego and an autonomous collective unconscious (Stephenson, 2017, p.2). Textbooks today are unlikely to mention the topic, although David Enoch's *Uncommon Psychiatric Syndromes*, now in its fifth edition, acquired a chapter on possession states in its second edition in 1979 (Enoch and Trethowan, 1979). If possession by demons or spirits is 'uncommon' in the practice of psychiatry in the Western world today, it is certainly not uncommon worldwide. Numerous case reports have been published of patients presenting with possession beliefs in a psychiatric context. This chapter will focus on a case study of a patient belonging to a spiritualist church and will make further reference to Christian, Muslim and Spiritist traditions.[1]

Alejo

I met Alejo very early on in my psychiatric training, and only a few years after I had qualified as a doctor. He was a middle-aged father of four teenaged children who had moved to the UK with his family from Columbia when he was still a child. He presented one Friday evening, in the accident and emergency department of the hospital where I was on call. I'm sure that a whole book could be written about presentations of patients with complex conditions who appear looking for help at the end of a working week, just as consultants and GPs are going home for the weekend. This was one such case, although it was his family that brought him to the hospital, and he was not referred by his GP. His presenting complaint was that he believed he was possessed by evil spirits.

Alejo had recently started experiencing violent moods and had occasionally been physically violent to others (although not so as to cause any serious injury). He had awoken in the night, agitated and saying, 'Something's in me! Get it out!' Both he and his wife said that they could smell rotting flesh in the bedroom. When morning came, he said that he wanted to see a priest – urgently. He went to see a priest that morning and asked him to exorcise the evil spirit, but the priest had not been able to help. I wish I had asked more about what exactly the priest did – but that was not something that seemed to matter to Alejo at the time. What did matter to him was that the priest hadn't been able to help. Having sought help unsuccessfully from religion, he was now turning to psychiatry.

Alejo had been attending a spiritualist church for two years and was playing with a Ouija board and tarot cards at home, in secret, against advice received from longer-standing members of the church. His sisters were involved in the same church, and one of them had been encouraging him in his attendance there and in his general involvement with spiritualism.

There was no past psychiatric history, but Alejo had a complicated family history. His mother and two other maternal relatives had received a diagnosis of Huntington's chorea. One of his uncles had already died of the condition. Alejo had done a lot of research on Huntington's chorea, but – somewhat incongruously – denied being worried that he might also be a carrier of the gene. Given the potentially serious implications for his own health

---

[1] For two case reports in the context of Judaism, see Somer, 2004. For two case studies in a Buddhist cultural context, see Eguchi, 1991. Studies in a Hindu context seem to be especially numerous. For a case study of a Hindu patient in India, see Basu et al., 2002. Chandrashekar et al. (1980) report a series of 30 patients in India, all but one of whom were Hindu. In a series of 201 psychiatric patients in India studied by Shidhaye and Vankar (2011), 92 per cent of whom were Hindus, 22 (10.5%) were identified as having experienced possession disorder (all of whom had been to see a traditional healer before going to a psychiatrist). In an interesting study in Sri Lanka, also mostly of Hindu subjects, 7 per cent (30) of 426 psychiatric patients, and 2 per cent (30) of 1,492 medical patients, were identified as having possession states. The possessing spirits did not necessarily match the religion of the patients, with Christians reporting possession by Hindu spirits, and vice versa.

and well-being, and that of his children, this seemed strange. It would have been much more natural and understandable if he had been deeply worried about the possibility of carrying the Huntington's gene. Given his age, it was entirely possible that – if he was a carrier for the gene – he was drawing close to the age at which the first symptoms might present. He was well aware that it was a cause of presenile dementia, severe neurological disability and premature death.

On mental state examination, Alejo wore a vacant expression, and his mood was somewhat flat. Despite this, he intermittently smiled at inappropriate points in the conversation. He reported hearing voices. The voices told him that he had a gift for mediumship. One voice, a 'good' voice, told him that his wife was a medium and another, a 'bad' voice, that he was a bad person. The voices were telling him what to do and told him that they were going to take him away from his body and that he would die. He was strongly convinced that he was possessed by an evil spirit (or spirits). Given his spiritualist beliefs, this was not necessarily thought to be delusional.

There was much debate amongst the clinical team about the most appropriate diagnosis. It was thought that his voices were not true hallucinations, and that his experiences of being told what to do by them did not amount to passivity phenomena. With hindsight, and with knowledge of research undertaken over the decades since (see Chapter 5), his hallucinations would fall into the category of those that were more thought-like, rather than auditory, but this does not appear to have much (or any) diagnostic significance. According to the thinking of the time, they could reasonably be judged to be pseudo-hallucinations. As to whether or not he was experiencing passivity phenomena, this in itself was also a very subjective judgement. Spiritually significant hallucinations may, more often than previously realised, include command hallucinations (Cook et al., 2022). The voices had been telling him not to eat, and he had consequently lost weight. It was not clear what else they might instruct him to do that might cause him (or others) harm.

Whilst Alejo was on the ward, he received a visit from a spiritualist healer and initially claimed that the spirits had been cast out. However, his mental state did not change significantly following this, and he continued to look emotionally bland and smiled inappropriately during conversation. When asked, he said that he would be pleased to receive a visit from a Christian minister, to further discuss the possibility of exorcism or deliverance, but did not actively pursue this, and the consultant in charge was against the idea.

Spiritualism

Spiritualism has its origins in Hydesville, New York, in 1848, in the home of John and Margaret Fox and their two youngest daughters, Kate and Margaret. There are different ways of telling the story, according to what one believes, or wants to believe. One narrative is that the two sisters devised a system of knocking sounds (which they secretly made, initially, using an apple on a string) as a means of communicating with an alleged spirit (Bullough, 1985; Pimple, 1995; Chapin, 2000; Weisberg, 2005). Public interest grew, and they attracted wide attention, as people were fascinated by the possibility of communication with deceased spirits. There was extensive empirical investigation of the alleged communications, which many interpreted as giving support to the theory that the knocking sounds could be explained on the basis of a deception. After many years the sisters admitted that it had all been a childish hoax, but then, a year later, they recanted their confession (for reasons which are also open to debate). The recantation opened the door for people to continue to believe in another possible narrative, according to which there actually had been genuine communication with the spirits of the deceased.

What we believe is powerfully shaped by what we want to believe. Clearly many in Hydesville, and farther afield, did want to continue to believe that it was possible to communicate with the dead. The empirical evidence, many believe, weighed against the spiritualist narrative, but scientific evidence is only a part of the story (whichever narrative you adopt). Faith is usually, if not always, based partly, or even primarily, upon other ways of knowing. What we think we know, in matters of spirituality and faith, is a complex mixture of reason, different kinds of evidence, personal experience and a desire to believe one thing rather than another. Something in this story caught the imagination of many, and the spiritualist movement continued to grow, especially during and after the First World War, but it later declined. In the 2001 Census, there were 32,000 identifiable spiritualists in the UK (Purdam et al., 2010).[2]

The philosophy of spiritualism comprises seven principles:

1. The Fatherhood of God
2. The Brotherhood of Man
3. The Communion of Saints and the Ministry of Angels
4. Continuous Existence of the Human Soul
5. Personal Responsibility
6. Compensation and Retribution hereafter for all the Good and Evil Deeds done on Earth
7. Eternal Progress open to Every Human Soul. (Walliss, 2001, p.131)

The crucial outworking of these principles, especially the third, is that physical death is not the end of human existence and that, through mediums, those who are deceased can continue to communicate with those who are alive on Earth. This can take place in passive and active ways. In the passive form, the medium is possessed by a spirit, thus providing the channel of communication with the spirit world. However, it is the active form that has become more common in contemporary spiritualism (Walliss, 2001, p.132), and possession seems to be reported rarely amongst spiritualists, at least in the UK (Rubinstein, 1984). When it does occur, blame is often attributed to the victim, for example because they are said to have become involved in circles (seances) without being sufficiently prepared to control the spirits that are contacted there (Rubinstein, 1984). Alejo appeared to be in just such a situation. He was apparently blamed for his own possession because he had not been heeding the warnings (e.g., against playing with Ouija boards) given by other members of his spiritualist church.

Possession States

Demon possession might seem like a very strange concept for psychiatry in the late twentieth or early twenty-first century in a very secular country such as the UK. However, in her groundbreaking studies of possession, the anthropologist Erika Bourguignon (1924–2015) found that possession beliefs were observed in 74 per cent of the 488 societies in her worldwide sample (Bourguignon, 1978). Whilst only 52 per cent of societies in North

---

[2] There was no category for spiritualism in the UK census form. However, amongst those that indicated that their religion was 'other' than the categories provided, there was an option to indicate religious affiliation, for those who wanted to do so.

America held such beliefs, the figure was 88 per cent in the Insular Pacific. Belief in possession is thus very common worldwide. However, as Bourguignon pointed out, it is not universal. From an anthropological perspective, in contrast to a theological one, it is a 'human invention' or a 'cultural artifact' (Bourguignon, 1978, p.502). Possession is widely acknowledged in almost all the world's major faith traditions. This does not mean that all Christians, or all Muslims or Jews or others, will necessarily believe in literal demonic entities. Evil, and a language of demonic and spiritual beings, finds a place within Islamic and Judeo-Christian scriptures and traditions but it is interpreted by theologians and by lay believers in a variety of ways, some of which ascribe ontological reality and some of which do not.

In *Ecstatic Religion: An Anthropological Study of Spirit Possession and Shamanism*, I. M. Lewis (1930–2014) explored the social functions of spirit possession and shamanism. Lewis's comparative study considered shamanism in Africa, Arctic Asia and South America, as well as Haitian voodoo and classical and Christian mysticism (Lewis, 1975). He distinguished between peripheral possession, in which the possessing spirits are amoral and originate outside the societies concerned, and in which those possessed (usually women) occupy peripheral positions within their societies, and main morality possession religions (or central possession religions) involving possession either by ancestral spirits or deities which, in either case, are strictly moralistic. Mediated by priests or shamans, possession here functions to maintain social and political order. Lewis saw psychiatry as a 'latent function' (Lewis, 1975, p.198) of shamanism. Like psychiatry, it identifies the social origins of mental disturbance, but it also concerns itself with illness and misfortune more widely: 'shamanism is more than psychiatry' (p.199). Psychiatry and psychoanalysis, for Lewis, were 'imperfect forms of shamanism' (p.199).

Bourguignon shared Lewis's interest in cultural interpretations of altered states of consciousness, but introduced a different classification of possession beliefs (Bourguignon, 1973, pp.28–29). Possession could be either sought or unsought, and associated with trance, or else not associated with trance (Bourguignon, 1976). To some extent accommodating the work of Lewis, Bourguignon and others, DSM-5 and ICD-11 both emphasise that a diagnosis of dissociative trance (300.15 in DSM-5) or possession trance disorder (6B63 in ICD-11) should not be made in the absence of significant distress or impairment. Possession/trance may often be a part of accepted cultural/religious practices and thus does not necessarily constitute pathology. William Dalrymple, for example, provides a vivid account of sought possession trance in modern India, in which ritual possession by Hindu deities functions to provide hope and address social injustice (Dalrymple, 2009, pp.29–55). In clinical practice, it is usually unsought possession that is the cause for concern, whether or not associated with trance. However, as Alejo's story illustrates, patients may have begun by seeking particular spiritual experiences and then find that things get out of control. Something that begins as 'sought' may lead to unsought and unwanted consequences.

For transcultural psychiatry, the challenge lays in managing the potential conflicts and tensions between a medical and a cultural worldview. Some possession states may resemble, or be associated with, a psychiatric diagnosis. Some psychiatric diagnoses may present with beliefs about spirit possession. Possession beliefs may serve to interpret signs and symptoms of underlying illness, especially mental illness. Roland Littlewood (2004) draws attention to the importance of sensitivity to local culture in such circumstances. If local cultural beliefs and norms are ignored, there is a danger that the clinician will lose the patient's or relatives' engagement with medical care, and that the patient's own insight into their condition will not properly be understood. If local culture is over-emphasised, there is a danger that a treatable diagnosis will be missed, that patients will not receive the medical support they need and that they may be exposed to idiosyncratic and potentially harmful local healing practices.

Littlewood has suggested that possession is 'arguably the most common culture-bound psychiatric syndrome' (Littlewood, 2004, p.8). As such, it would appear most often to be recognised not so much as an illness (although it is seen as this by some) as an 'idiom of distress' (Nichter, 1981; Hinton and Lewis-Fernandez, 2010). Ruma Bose (1997), for example, presents case studies of two young Bangladeshis living in London identified as experiencing *upridosh* – where their unusual behaviour is attributed to jinn, or spirits. In the one case, a girl worried about her examinations in her last year at school became initially paranoid and excited, but then stopped talking, eating and drinking. An Islamic healer advised that this was owing to jinn possession. She subsequently woke at night, screaming and saying that she had seen Shaitan (Satan). In the other case, a 15-year-old boy whose father had died was sent to an Islamic boarding school, away from his family. Alone in his room, he felt himself thrown off his bed by a powerful force, which he identified as Hawa (wind) by which he believed he was possessed. When he returned home, he felt strange and fearful. His behaviour changed and he became mute and stopped eating, then began shouting and became overactive. In both cases, the condition was dealt with by a combination of intervention by an Islamic healer and psychiatric treatment from local mental health services. Bose speculates that an appropriate diagnosis might be of a situational reaction, or acute and transient psychosis, but such idioms of distress do not fit neatly into standardised psychiatric categories.

There are criticisms of the medicalisation of possession in the diagnostic systems of psychiatry, pointing out that it is often viewed non-pathologically in local contexts and that it is an unhelpful way of converting distress into disease (Padmanabhan, 2017). In a mixed-methods study of 22 possessed and 16 non-possessed women in a village in Nepal (Sapkota et al., 2014), it was found that possessed women had higher rates of traumatic events and scored higher on symptoms of mental disorder in relation to the control group. However, qualitative interviews revealed that the possessed women did not associate possession with mental illness but saw it, rather, as a means of communication with spirits. Possession thus functioned as an idiom of distress. In a study of domestic abuse and trauma in Malaysia (Sahdan et al., 2021), possession functioned as both an explanation and a justification for abuse, thus, in this case, serving as a cultural idiom for the experiences of both perpetrator and victim.

A shaman is an inspired priest (Lewis, 1975, pp.49–57) who voluntarily becomes possessed, as a 'master of spirits' (p.56; c.f., Kharitidi's *Master of Lucid Dreams*, 2001), in order to provide a mediation between divine spirits and human beings. Some of the functions of shamanism (but not all) are thus shared with mediums. Alejo's problems appear to have been at this interface but, whereas the medium and the shaman are in control of the spirits that possess them, Alejo clearly was not.

Demonic Struggles

Belief that one is possessed by a demon or spirit represents a particular example of a broader category of demonic struggles. In order to find oneself involved in such a struggle, it is necessary to make demonic attributions, defined by Pargament and Exline (2022) as deciding 'that demonic entities are playing a role in a situation, either by causing or influencing events' (p.276). The language here may be of demons specifically, or it may be of the Devil or Satan, of spirits of various sorts, curses, witchcraft or evil of other kinds. The word 'demonic' is used here to refer to all of these kinds of evil, although of course they are theologically diverse. In Alejo's case, his preferred language was that of 'spirits', deriving from his association with the spiritualist church.

According to Pargament and Exline (2022, pp.276–283), demonic attributions are a necessary but not sufficient component of demonic struggles. Demonic attributions are shaped by worldview and, thus, for most people worldwide, religious belief. They require some kind of belief that a supernatural adversary of some sort exists, and that this adversary has influence in the world. Assuming that these beliefs are in place, they may further be fostered by social engagement with groups that promote these beliefs in active ways, and especially the more fundamentalist forms of religions such as Christianity or Islam. However, beyond all of this, there do also seem to be important individual differences in disposition when it comes to making demonic attributions.

In terms of personal disposition, for example, an intuitive rather than an analytic cognitive style may make someone more likely to believe in demons, as well as more likely to hold religious beliefs more widely (Pennycook et al., 2012). Significant life events may also be important (e.g., witnessing an act of immense evil, such as genocide), but perhaps more usually some people may put themselves in the way of repeated experiences that may predispose to demonic attributions. For example, they may play with tarot cards or Ouija boards (as Alejo did), or engage in malevolent forms of witchcraft, or attend seances. In addition to all of this, mental illness may contribute to individual propensity to attribute events and experiences to the Devil or the demonic.

For demonic attributions to be made in respect of specific events, they need to be accessible, plausible, meaningful and motivating (Pargament and Exline, 2022, pp.280–282). Negative events are more likely to be attributed to Satan than positive events (Lupfer et al., 1996), and yet Satan may be understood as acting more through people's thoughts and actions, with a lack of clarity about how exactly he may influence the occurrence of the events themselves (Ray et al., 2015). Belief in evil forces may be motivated by a search for meaning, especially amongst those of high religiosity (Routledge et al., 2016), and may serve to reduce the sense in which God is seen to be to blame for the evil that happens in the world (Beck and Taylor, 2008).

For demonic attributions to become demonic struggles, Pargament and Exline (2022, p.282) suggest, there needs to be a perceived threat. There might be an appraisal suggesting that the Devil is out to cause personal harm, or that if the person accedes to what they believe the Devil is leading them to do then God might cause them harm. When personal resources are depleted, through tiredness, exhaustion, confusion or emotional distress, the sense of struggle may be enhanced. Lack of social support, a sense of personal guilt, poor self-esteem or depression may also all increase the sense of threat.

Differential Diagnosis

In their 1979 chapter on possession states and allied syndromes, Enoch and Trethowan (1979, pp.160–190) considered that ideas of possession are likely to be owing to either psychosis (principally, schizophrenia or depression) or else perhaps obsessive-compulsive disorder. By the fifth edition of the book, in 2021, this list had expanded to include organic psychosis, dissociative identity disorder, personality disorder and bereavement reactions (Enoch et al., 2021, p.255).

In a 1993 article on differential diagnosis of possession states, alongside an account of culturally normative possession states, Philip Coons identified possible psychopathological forms as including multiple personality disorder, trance possession disorder, psychosis and culture-bound psychiatric syndromes such as amok (in Malaysia), piblokto (in Alaska) and whitigo (amongst the Cree and Ojibwa native Americans). Curiously, Coons also included demon possession in Christianity as a form of psychopathology (Coons, 1993). He justifies this on the basis that, in contrast to other cultural examples of trance possession, it is unsought. However, trance possession in other cultural groups may also be unsought, and – if Coons believed it to be pathological – it is not clear why he did not include it as a culture-bound syndrome.

The empirical literature, which includes few systematic studies, and almost none with large sample sizes or control groups, reveals some interesting variations of emphasis in regard to the range and kinds of diagnosis that might present as possession. There are now a very large number of published case studies.

During et al. (2011) identified 28 papers published globally, from 1988 to 2010, giving reports of a total of 402 cases of dissociative trance disorder (DTD), 69 per cent of which could be classified as possession type. Amongst those with possession disorder, 56 per cent reported hallucinations, and only 20 per cent amnesia. The authors identify nine 'major aetiological frameworks' (list drawn from p.238):

1. psychosocial stressors
2. trauma (including sexual abuse, war, violence in childhood, etc.)
3. underlying psychiatric conditions (including psychosis, personality disorder, neurosis, etc.)
4. cultural factors
5. communication theory (expression of difficulties experienced by the oppressed)
6. gain-seeking (diversely including mediumship, economic/other gain, positive labelling)
7. dissociative states
8. hysteria
9. acculturation (following migration or conversion).

The believed possessing agents included various kinds of deities and angels (43%), deceased human spirits (29%), demons and other malevolent spirits (jinn, zar, etc.) (18%), animals (5%), the Devil (4%) and – in only one patient – a local saint. The authors conclude that DTD is a 'global idiom of distress, probably underdiagnosed in Western countries' (During et al., 2011, p.235).

There have been a number of publications,[3] from around the world, reporting on patients, like Alejo, presenting to psychiatric services with beliefs that they were possessed. Typically, the diagnoses made include, most commonly, psychoses (especially schizophrenia) and hysteria or (to use the current terminology) dissociative disorders. In some cases, an organic disorder is diagnosed (e.g., confusion/delirium). Depression, borderline personality disorder and anxiety also appear, so that almost the entire spectrum of psychiatric diagnoses may apparently present in this way, at least in some places, some of the time.

---

[3] See Yap, 1960; Teja et al., 1970; Varma et al., 1970; Whitwell and Barker, 1980; Iida, 1989; Goff et al., 1991; Gaw et al., 1998.

An association with early trauma is noted in the more recent literature. Hecker et al. (2015) identified 21 articles on spirit possession, in low- and middle-income countries, published between 1994 and 2013. They were able to collate data on 917 patients with possession trance disorders. They identified a strong relationship with trauma, with especially high rates in post-war countries in Africa. With the help of local traditional and spiritual healers in the Democratic Republic of the Congo, Hecker et al. (2016) identified 73 people who had experienced pathological spirit possession. Possession symptom severity correlated with lifetime post-traumatic stress disorder (PTSD) symptom severity and depressive symptoms.

Goff et al. (1991) studied 61 patients with a history of chronic psychosis, 25 of whom had delusions of possession. The latter group more commonly reported a history of childhood sexual abuse and higher scores for dissociative experiences. In a study of 628, mostly Muslim, women in Turkey (Sar et al., 2014), 13 gave a history of possession. Women with a history of trauma were more likely to report possession than those without.

The psychiatric diagnosis which has caused more debate than any other in relation to possession states is that of dissociative identity disorder (DID). It has been argued that some historical accounts of demon possession might in fact have been cases of DID (Van Der Hart et al., 1996) and that DID patients not infrequently report possession related experiences (Ross, 2011). However, the association may be culturally dependent (Adityanjee et al., 1989; Gingrich, 2006) and when modern-day sufferers of DID have been subjected to exorcism, adverse psychological and spiritual outcomes have sometimes been documented (e.g., Bowman, 1993). In DSM-5, there is reference to 'possession-form' cases of DID, in which certain alters present as spirits:

> Possession-form identities in dissociative identity disorder typically manifest as behaviours that appear as if a 'spirit', supernatural being, or outside person has taken control, such that the individual begins speaking or acting in a distinctly different manner. For example, an individual's behavior may give the appearance that her identity has been replaced by the 'ghost' of a girl who committed suicide in the same community years before, speaking and acting as though she were still alive. (American Psychiatric Association, 2013, p.293)

The text of DSM-5 goes on to emphasise that 'the majority of possession states around the world are normal' and do not meet the criteria for the diagnosis. However, critics argue that this pathologisation of an essentially normal cultural phenomenon creates an impossible task for clinicians attempting to distinguish between cultural and pathological manifestations of spiritual distress and that it represents a reductionistic and political appropriation of possession as a primarily medical concern (e.g., Stephenson, 2017, pp.94–96). Criteria for distinguishing pathological from non-pathological manifestations of possession trance phenomena (within the scope of which DID falls) include culturally accepted practice, the presence or absence of psychiatric history or other personal distress, and lack of training in relevant ritual practices (Cardeña, 2023, p.426). On this basis, Alejo might be identified as having at least two out of three indicators of pathology (personal distress and lack of training in communicating with spirits), but it is not clear that these criteria are likely to be of help in many cases. Dissociative identity disorder is known to be commonly associated with co-morbidity and distress, and most people who present as possessed conform in some way or another to cultural expectations. Ritual practices, in most cases of demon possession or other unsought forms of possession, apply more to those who respond by way of offering exorcism or healing, rather than to the person who is possessed.

True vs False Possession

In a review of 53 documented cases of spirit/demon possession between 1890 and 2023, Escolà-Gascón et al. (2023) calculated that the probability of encountering a case of possession that is scientifically unexplained is less than 2 per cent. Whilst they do distinguish between 'unexplained' and 'inexplicable', it is not entirely clear what 'unexplained' means in the context of their study. One suspects that the true figure, across the published literature, is likely to be significantly less than 2 per cent.

In general, it is unsurprising that psychiatrists tend to see possession states as psychopathological and anthropologists as culturally normative. However, in the theological and religious literature there is debate concerning the distinction between true possession and false or pseudo-possession. For example, Michael Perry (1933–2015), a Church of England priest with considerable experience in this field, and drawing on the experience of the Christian Deliverance Study Group in the UK, distinguished between 'possession syndrome', by which he seemed to mean any psychiatric condition with a clinical presentation including belief in being possessed, and true possession, which he believed to be owing to 'the activity of an evil spirit' (Perry, 1996, p.118). Perhaps this is what one would expect a priest to say. However, some medical writers have also emphasised the importance of making such distinctions.

Jean Lhermitte (1877–1959), a French neurologist interested in the relationship between theology and medicine, made such a distinction in his book *Diabolical Possession, True and False* (Lhermitte, 1963), published originally in French (as *Vrais et Faux Possédés*) in 1956. Some years later, M. Scott Peck (1936–2005), an American psychiatrist, in *Glimpses of the Devil* (Peck, 2005), described two cases which he believed were examples of true possession. More recently, Richard Gallagher (2022), another American psychiatrist and a member of the International Association of Exorcists, who has quite probably seen more cases of possession than any other psychiatrist worldwide, describes his experience of what he believes to have been true possessions. Unsurprisingly, his views have been seen as very controversial in the press and on social media. All of these doctors were/are Christians.

Possession states take on a different emphasis and perspective in other faith traditions, but the same question arises, albeit in different forms. Does the scientific and medical worldview of the psychiatrist leave open any possibility of something that might be called 'true' possession? Muslim patients widely believe in the existence of jinn. In the Qur'an, jinn are said to have been made from the 'fire of scorching wind' (27:15) or 'fire free of smoke' (55.15). Although many Muslims believe that jinn may be the cause of mental illness (Lim et al., 2018), there is debate as to whether or not this is actually what the Qur'an teaches (Islam and Campbell, 2014). In the medical literature, the widely discussed question concerns how popular belief in jinn might be reconciled with a medical diagnosis. The possibility of true jinn possession is rarely voiced in medical texts,[4] although in one recent study it has been claimed that true jinn possession can be detected by thermal imaging (Rahman et al., 2021a). It is generally acknowledged that patients' views on jinn should not be contradicted, but that a form of words is needed which allows patients, medical professionals and imams to work together (Ascoli et al., 2014).

---

[4] But, for exceptions, see Bayer and Shunaigat, 2002 and Khalifa and Hardie, 2005.

In Spiritism (not to be confused with spiritualism), where the spirits concerned are understood as discarnate human spirits rather than demons, and the term 'obsession' is used in preference to 'possession', spirit release therapy, or disobsession, is understood as a spiritual treatment for some forms of mental disorder. Conventional psychiatric treatments are provided alongside disobsession in many psychiatric hospitals in Brazil (Moreira-Almeida and Lotufo Neto, 2005; Lucchetti et al., 2012). Within this paradigm, the differential diagnosis seems primarily to be concerned with distinguishing conditions that are caused by obsessions from those that are not (Moreira-Almeida and Lotufo Neto, 2005). If the condition is caused by an obsession, then the 'diagnosis' becomes a matter of discerning the nature of the problem experienced by the obsessing spirit. For example, Greenfield (2004) describes the disobsession of a (male) patient whose problem was said to be owing to an abortion that he had had in a previous (female) lifetime. The obsessing spirit, in this case, was said to be the discarnate spirit of the aborted fetus.

In broader terms, the diagnosis of DID is deeply problematic in relation to proposed distinctions between true and false possession. How might any case of 'true' possession be distinguished from possession-form DID, other than by the alleged supernatural phenomena (such as levitation or speaking in languages not previously learnt) to which theological authorities often refer (Cook, 2025b)? Even in these cases, there is often scope for sceptics to question the evidence or present alternative explanations. The Jungian concept of autonomous unconscious complexes (or other theoretical explanations of how alters are generated) might be said to be a different way of talking about the same thing, simply moving the conversation to questions of ontology rather than veracity. As discussed in Chapter 4, what is really needed, rather than a political appropriation of possession states by one discipline or another, is a critical dialogue between the disciplines of theology and psychiatry.

Therapy

Exline et al. (2021) have proposed that there are three lenses through which to frame demonic struggles in therapy: mental illness, psychological and supernatural. Each has its own strengths and limitations, but Exline et al. draw attention to the unfamiliarity of the supernatural lens to most mental health professionals and to some of the potentially adverse outcomes if the supernatural lens is adopted without reference to the other two. Clearly, the treatment provided for mental illness will depend upon the diagnosis. This is not the place to explore current approaches to treatment for all of the diagnoses mentioned in the section of this chapter on 'Differential Diagnosis'. However, whatever the diagnosis may be, and whatever the best current evidence and standards of good psychiatric practice would dictate as appropriate treatment for patients with such a diagnosis, treatment planning would properly involve spiritual care as part of a patient-centred approach to caring for the whole person.

The psychological lens, whether or not there is also a psychiatric diagnosis, offers important insights not only in terms of psychological therapies but also in terms of understanding the part that spirituality/religion play when a patient believes that they are oppressed or possessed by evil spiritual forces. There is a complex relationship between the spiritual and the psychological in which it is virtually impossible to separate the one from the other. Beliefs about demons may be a cause of anxiety, fear and paranoia, but, equally, anxiety and fear, in a particular spiritual/religious context, might cause someone to believe that they are under demonic attack. Spiritual and religious worldviews can serve a variety of psychological purposes. On the one hand, they may seem to make the world a more predictable place; they may provide emotional security, a moral framework and a sense of meaning and purpose in life. On the other hand, they may serve as psychological defences against uncertainty, anxiety and guilt in such a way as to obstruct conscious exploration of complex moral and emotional dilemmas. Projection of evil on to demonic forces may be a way of avoiding taking personal responsibility for the evil within or, as Jung would have it, the shadow side of the human psyche.

Pargament and Exline (2022, pp.292–297) suggest that an exploration of basic beliefs about evil and a psychological examination of demonic attributions should be followed by a re-examination of core beliefs. I think that this is a good model, but I do wonder how many therapists have the necessary combination of spiritual and psychological skills (as Pargament and Exline themselves clearly do) to undertake such a therapeutic task effect-ively, sensitively and respectfully when faced with a patient from an unfamiliar faith tradition. One possibility might be to collaborate with clergy, chaplains or other spiritual advisers in order to address spiritual and psychological issues jointly together. However, as Exline et al. acknowledge (2021, pp.221–222), not all therapists may be happy to do this, especially in relation to beliefs around evil and the demonic. Furthermore, this may raise significant professional boundary issues (see Chapter 8), especially where a therapist may feel that it is the nature of the underlying beliefs and attributions that needs to change and that these same beliefs and attributions may be the very ones that are reaffirmed by clergy, or by the faith community to which the patient belongs. Some of the professional issues that arise in a Christian context are further explored by me elsewhere (Cook, 2024b).

Exorcism

The 'obvious' solution to demon possession, at least in Western cultural terms, is expulsion of the evil entity – exorcism. This seemingly obvious approach, sometimes referred to as anthropemic (a vomiting or expulsion of the evil other) is not the only conceivable response and is not the universal norm. Psychologically, and culturally, there is also the option to invoke, integrate or appropriate that which is psychologically other, an option sometimes referred to as adorcism. In some cultures, this is the preferred approach (as, for example, in zar possession in Sudan) and in Jungian analytical psychology the acknowledgement and (as far as possible) integration of unconscious psychological complexes may be the preferred therapeutic goal (Stephenson, 2017). I confess that I never thought of this when working with Alejo, but, equally, outside those cultural contexts which affirm adorcism, or the therapeutic space of a Jungian analysis, the idea of welcoming into the psyche that which is identified as evil is psychologically and theologically counter-intuitive, potentially spir-itually harmful and unlikely to be seen as attractive to most patients or clinicians. The question therefore arises as to whether and how, psychologically and spiritually, exorcism might be a helpful therapeutic response.

Julian Leff (1975), a distinguished social psychiatrist, has suggested that exorcism might be considered an 'exotic' psychiatric treatment. Alejo's consultant clearly did not share this view, or else felt that it was too 'exotic' to be professionally recommended. Considering exorcism alongside various other traditional approaches to treating what we would consider to be psychiatric disorders, Leff points to the example of Jesus exorcising the Gerasene demoniac (as recorded in the Christian Gospels attributed to Mark and Luke) as illustrative of the benefits of traditional treatments more widely:

In Jesus's healing technique we find all the elements that are common to the procedures used by native healers throughout the world when dealing with mental illness. He commands the devils to leave the possessed sufferer, he transfers them into the bodies of animals, and the animals are subsequently killed. There is the additional element of water to wash away the evil spirits. (Leff, 1975, p.126)

Leff acknowledges that thousands of years of tradition, and worldwide practice, are no guarantee of efficacy. Nonetheless, he continues, 'the spread through time and space of exorcism ceremonies for psychiatric conditions suggests that at least they are catering to some aspect of the patients' disturbed state of mind. One important feature seems to be the provision of an explanation that is acceptable in terms of the beliefs of the patient and his relatives' (p.126). Leff concludes that, although Western psychiatry has displaced many traditional healing practices, we should not dismiss them out of hand; there remains a need for them. His reflections are a helpful corrective to a tendency towards a very restrictive, reductionistic and overly scientific approach to contemporary psychiatry. However, I'm left wondering, how – in contemporary Western psychiatry – do we retain explanations that are 'acceptable in terms of the beliefs of the patient and his relatives' and at the same time address the complex interplay between what we now understand as the biopsychosocial model and its spiritual concomitants? How does the encounter between exorcism and evidence-based practice play out in our cultural context?

It is immediately necessary to acknowledge that we do not have the systematic controlled trials of exorcism that we really need to formulate reliable, evidence-based, scientific answers to our questions (Rosik, 1997). However, this is not to say that there is no evidence, only that the evidence takes the form of individual case studies and uncontrolled studies with small sample sizes.

Perhaps the most salutary story in relation to the exorcism of someone who was suffering from mental illness, at least in the UK, is that of Michael Taylor.[5] In 1974, Michael Taylor was subjected to an all-night exorcism by the vicar of his Anglican parish church, near Barnsley in Yorkshire, assisted by the local Methodist minister and several others. On the following morning, he murdered his wife, Christine, and was found wandering naked, covered in blood which he said was 'the blood of Satan'. At his trial, he was found not guilty of murder, by reason of insanity, and sent to Broadmoor Hospital. The psychiatrist called as an expert witness, Hugo Milne, expressed the view that the murder would not have happened but for the exorcism. Church of England guidelines introduced following this event stressed the importance of 'collaboration with the resources of medicine' when engaging in such ministry. More recent guidelines have updated this basic advice, but they present difficult questions about how this should properly happen in practice (Cook, 2024b).

Even if the consequences are usually less extreme than this, ineffective and negative outcomes to exorcism have been reported in cases of DID (Bowman, 1993; Fraser, 1993; Rosik, 1997) and schizophrenia (Hale and Pinninti, 1994; Tajima-Pozo et al., 2011). Exorcism has been reported to effect change of gender identity (Barlow et al., 1977) and sexual orientation (Ross and Stålström, 1979), something which would now undoubtedly contravene the cross-professional consensus that conversion therapies for sexual orientation and gender identity are unethical (UK Council for Psychotherapy, 2014). However,

---

[5] I'm currently working on a new article on this subject, with Gwen Adshead.

positive outcomes have been reported in relation to depression and schizophrenia (Maniam, 1987), and DID (Bull et al., 1998). Al-Krenawi and Graham (1997) report the treatment of a Bedouin patient for whom exorcism and mental health care were successfully combined.

In a study of 15 patients with DID (Bull et al., 1998), a positive response to exorcism was associated with eight factors:

1. patient permission
2. noncoercion
3. active participation of the patient
4. understanding of DID dynamics by the exorcist
5. implementation of the exorcism within the context of psychotherapy
6. compatibility of the procedure with the patient's spiritual beliefs
7. incorporation of the patient's belief system
8. encouragement of patient self-independence regarding exorcism.

(p.188, numbering added)

It might seem surprising that such basic considerations as patient consent and non-coercion must be explicitly identified as necessary for a good outcome, but it would seem that they were not always in place in some of the studies with negative outcomes. The contextualisation of exorcism within a course of psychological therapy, and the need for an understanding of the mental health condition by the person conducting the exorcism, would also seem to be fundamental, and yet it was exactly the absence of such considerations that led to the tragic outcome in the case of Michael Taylor.

Whatever one makes of these conflicting reports, the initial diagnosis is not always clear and, in the cases of allegedly positive outcomes, is often in doubt. In a study of 17 people experiencing exorcism in a Nigerian-based Pentecostal church in London, who seem to have had generally positive outcomes, the difficulty in distinguishing between spiritual experiences of possession and psychosis was noted (Rowan and Dwyer, 2015). In a case study of a Bedouin patient who responded well to exorcism, the original diagnosis of schizophrenia was considered mistaken (Al-Krenawi and Graham, 1997).

Alejo: On Reflection

As a young psychiatrist, I couldn't really work out what diagnosis was appropriate, given Alejo's presentation. At the case conference, after many possibilities were considered, a senior colleague commented, 'Perhaps he is possessed!' I wonder now if he may have been right, although – if he was – I would understand this differently now than I did then. Alejo's presentation conformed, as far as I can tell, to expectations of what possession might look like within the spiritualist church to which he belonged. Whatever theological questions this might raise as to the ontological nature of evil, the psychological reality that possession represents would have been more than enough to account for his affective state and perceptual experiences. It was a very effective idiom of distress, but what exactly was the nature of that distress?

Alejo's demonic attributions were shaped by the religious community to which he belonged, and probably further reinforced by an intuitive cognitive style as well as by the experiences that he repeatedly exposed himself to through experimentation with Ouija boards and tarot cards. The threat that turned Alejo's attributions into demonic struggles might be understood at a number of levels. Although largely unacknowledged, the threat to life and family that his genetic diagnosis represented was considerable. In addition to this, his faith community seems to have put him in fear of the adverse consequences likely to follow from his use of Ouija and Tarot. Whereas this might, in theory, have been resolved through exorcism or spiritual healing of some kind, the genetic threat that he faced was not amenable to exorcism of any kind (at least, not within the bounds of genetic technology at that time). Nonetheless, I wish that we had established better communication with Alejo's faith community in order to find ways of turning their criticisms of him into a positive and supportive social influence and explored further the possibility of some kind of exorcism as a means of releasing him from the perceived spiritual and psychological threat. Positive and negative spiritual coping are closely related, and the same factors that promote the latter can potentially be recruited, in suitably modified form, to support the former.

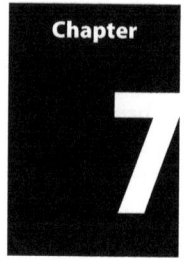

Prayer, Mindfulness and Silence

If positive and negative spiritual coping are two sides of a coin, with power respectively to improve or impair mental health outcomes, the question arises as to whether and how spiritual/religious concerns might be incorporated into psychiatric treatments in such a way as to improve outcomes. Much attention has been given to this question in research and clinical practice in recent years and a range of spiritually (or religiously) integrated treatments have been proposed, researched and incorporated into clinical practice. Some of these were considered in the second edition of *Spirituality and Psychiatry*, including mindfulness, forgiveness therapies, compassion-focussed therapies and religiously integrated cognitive behavioural therapy (CBT). Others occupy a space outside of formal psychiatric practice but are nonetheless highly important for psychiatrists to be aware of, notably the spiritual but not religious (SBNR) programme of recovery offered by Alcoholics Anonymous and other 12-step organisations.

The intention in this chapter is not to review the scientific and clinical evidence relating to these interventions, as that has been done elsewhere (e.g., Cook and Powell, 2022). Rather, the plan is to consider examples of some of the ways in which psychological therapies and spiritual/religious practices become entangled. These psycho-spiritual entanglements may potentially be either harmful or beneficial to the patient, and so it is important to be aware of them in treatment planning. The aim should be to ensure that they are utilised, where appropriate, to the benefit of both psychological recovery and spiritual growth.

A complete exploration of this interdisciplinary field would be a huge undertaking and so just three aspects of interest will be considered here by way of example of what might be more broadly important. Prayer in clinical practice has been professionally highly controversial, and yet prayer (corporate or personal) also features in the scientific research literature as a spiritual practice associated with good mental health outcomes. Mindfulness, a spiritual practice extracted from Buddhist tradition, but having much in common with contemplative practices in other religious traditions, has been extensively researched and is increasingly incorporated into the provisions of mental health service delivery and clinical treatment planning. Finally, silence, a spiritual practice identifiable within many faith traditions, and a phenomenon of interest in psychotherapy, will be considered as an under-researched and under-utilised common ground between the psychological and the spiritual in clinical practice.

Prayer

Prayer has been described as the 'central phenomenon of religion' (Heiler, 1932). Daily prayer is common practice around the world, albeit, in an analysis of 102 countries by the

Pew Research Center, it is less common in the UK than in any other country (Evans, 2024). In the USA, 44 per cent of respondents say that they pray daily (Pew Research Center, 2025), which seems to be about average worldwide. Daily prayer is particularly common in Islamic countries, with rates of 96 per cent in Afghanistan and 87 per cent in Iran (Pew Research Center, 2018, p.57). In Hindu-majority India, 75 per cent pray daily. However, prayer is practised even in secular societies (Bänziger et al., 2008a, 2008b) and a significant minority amongst the so-called religious nones are known to pray (Bullivant, 2017; Levin et al., 2022). Prayer is also practised by the SBNR (Simmons, 2021).

What is prayer? This seemingly simple question is amenable to a wide range of answers, even when confining it to one religion, such as Christianity. Philip and Carol Zaleski, in their history of prayer, have suggested that it is 'something like this: *prayer is action that communicates between human and divine realms*' (Zaleski and Zaleski, 2005, p.5, original emphasis preserved). Ann and Barry Ulanov, in their book on the psychology of prayer, writing from a Jungian perspective, have proposed that it is best understood as 'primary speech', arising out of our ability to put into words, and to listen to, our true selves (Ulanov and Ulanov, 1985). Whilst this may seem to open up the scope of prayer beyond what many would consider to be its proper theological ground, it should not be forgotten that images of God and self are interrelated, both having their origins in the human psyche (see Chapter 4). Thomas Merton, a Christian monk, encapsulated the entanglement succinctly as 'finding ourselves in God's truth' (Merton, 1969, p.92).

Prayer is motivated by desire, but the theological subject and object of prayer are easily confused. At first glance, prayer focusses on what we want (God to do). However, the act of prayer presents the person praying with questions about what it is that they really want – thus drawing him/her into what the Ulanovs would call primary speech. God, of course, does not need to be told what we want, or need, but in the process of asking we are invited to enlarge our self-knowledge. We are drawn, if we have the willingness and courage to be drawn, into articulating what we really want, and this almost always turns out to be something other than what we first imagined.[1] Unlike the depth psychologies, this prayerful process of increasing self-knowledge is not person-(or self-)centred; it is theocentric. Thus, we end up discovering that prayer is not really about what we desire but about God's desire for us. As Søren Kierkegaard (1813–1855), a Danish theologian and philosopher, cogently observed, 'prayer does not change God, but it changes the one who offers it' (Kierkegaard, 1961, p.44).

The precise nature of prayer will thus be bound up, on the one hand, with theologies of prayer (which, for clinical purposes, include primarily the ordinary theologies of those who pray) and, on the other hand, the biopsychosocial nature of the praying human being. Our prayers will be shaped both by what we believe and by who we are in our essential nature. Clearly, psychiatrists are most concerned with how this all pans out when psychopathology distorts the process. However, in order to properly understand the psychopathological distortions, it is necessary first to understand prayer as a part of daily life for many people worldwide and – in its broader conceptions (such as that proposed by the Ulanovs) – as a fundamental aspect of human nature.

---

[1] The relationship between prayer and desire is helpfully explored at greater length in chapter 2 of Ulanov and Ulanov, 1985.

Varieties of Prayer

As one would expect, the theology and the practice of prayer vary significantly between, and even within, religious traditions. There are major differences between Eastern and Western religions, with the former focussed more on prayer as a means to experience unification and the latter on relationship with God (Ladd et al., 2018). There are difficulties with language, with the word 'prayer' being more commonly employed in relation to Western religions and a variety of other terms and practices being used in the East. For example, words such as *bhakti* (loving devotion to particular manifestations of the divine), *puja* (worship in which offerings are made to a deity), or *darshana* (viewing the image of a deity) might be more commonly employed in Eastern traditions such as Hinduism.

There are also major points of misunderstanding, difference and controversy, as in attitudes to 'idols', which are valued as aids to prayer in Hinduism but strictly prohibited in the Abrahamic faiths. Indeed, it is debatable whether or not the word 'idol' is appropriate, such is the depth of controversy, and perhaps a more appropriate term would be 'icon' (Knott, 2016, pp.49–51). Icons in turn are controversial within Christianity, with many protestants believing that they are simply idols, and many Catholics and Orthodox finding that they are windows into another reality, not a focus in themselves.

Given these theological and religious differences, it is doubtful whether a scientific literature that has heavily focussed on the Judeo-Christian tradition can have been sufficiently sensitive to the kinds of methodological issues that could confound research on prayer. However, there is a scientific recognition that prayer is not a monolithic phenomenon, and it may be helpful here to consider briefly some of the approaches that have been taken to differentiate amongst different forms and practices of prayer in scientific research.

Based on telephone interviews with 560 residents of Akron, Ohio, Poloma and Pendleton (1989) identified four types of prayer: meditative, ritualist, petitionary and colloquial. Meditative prayer was said to be concerned with intimacy and relationship with God and was non-verbal. The other three types were all more active and verbal. Ritual prayer was concerned with recitation of prayers from liturgy or memory, petitionary with requests to God on behalf of self or others, and colloquial with less specific forms of conversation with God. Unsurprisingly, Poloma and Pendleton's Prayer Types Scale was later found not to have validity in non-Christian (Jewish and Muslim) subject samples, although it did appear to be possible to devise revised subscales specifically for use in each religious group (Black et al., 2015).

Bänziger et al. (2008a), in a study of 1,008 Dutch adults, also identified four varieties of prayer: petitionary, religious, meditative and impulsive. Religious and petitionary praying were the more traditionally theological kinds of prayer, both directed towards God, the former being more concerned with relationship with God, and the latter with specific requests for God to intervene, or else giving thanks. Meditative and impulsive prayer, in contrast, were described as more focussed within the psyche of the individual and typical of prayer in a secularised society. The terminology is slightly confusing in that 'meditative' might appear to imply the contemplative practices found in many traditional religious contexts. However, in this study, the meditative focus was inwards, non-theological and personal. Similarly, the impulsive category, although in many ways like petitionary prayer, was non-theological and more of a catharsis or 'pouring out of one's heart', with no requests being made for intervention.

In a study of a random sample of 1,248 adults in the USA, Laura Upenieks (2023) developed a typology based on why people pray. Most of the sample were Christian, 11 per cent were Jewish and 18 per cent non-affiliated. Again, four categories were identified: prayer *efficacy* was understood in relation to beliefs that prayer solves problems, *devotional* prayer was concerned with praise of God and prayer for others, prayer for *support* was in relation to matters such as health and finance, and prayer *expectancy* related to whether or not God answers prayer. These categories are not mutually exclusive and represent a dimensional, rather than a categorical, approach to studying prayer. Two-thirds of the sample agreed (at least to some extent) that prayer is the best way to solve world problems, and three-quarters that it is the best way to solve personal problems. Slightly more than three-quarters of the sample (77 per cent) agreed, at least to some extent, that God answers prayer.

In the taxonomy of religious health interventions developed by Patel et al. (2022), prayer appears under two main headings – intercessory and personal. These in turn are each broken down into four subcategories. The intercessory forms are very similar in description to petitionary prayer as described by Bänziger et al. (2008a); the personal forms are loosely similar to the religious type (although here also explicitly including more theologically contemplative and reflective practices).

A variety of other instruments have been developed in order to study, for example, such things as prayer experiences (Dein and Littlewood, 2008) and prayer importance (Tatala and Wojtasiński, 2021). One of the most comprehensive prayer questionnaires, which includes 11 prayer scales (that variously address sociality of prayer, prayer topics, and beliefs about God and the affective valence of prayer), is that used in the Baylor Religion Survey (Froese et al., 2024).

Prayer Preferences

Even within the same faith tradition, different people pray differently. For example, amongst 1,476 recently ordained Anglican clergy in the UK, significant correlations were found between prayer preferences and psychological type (assessed using the Keirsey Temperament sorter, on the basis of Jungian type theory) (Francis and Robbins, 2008). Introverts (I) preferred to pray alone and in silence, whereas extraverts (E) preferred praying vocally with groups of others. Sensing (S) types preferred traditional prayers, with an emphasis on use of pictures, hymns and prayer posture, whereas intuitive (N) types focussed much more on use of the imagination, on mystery and on the complexity of life. Thinking (T) prayer employed theological reflection and the use of reason, whereas feeling (F) prayer emphasised empathy with others, intimacy with God, compassion and relational concerns. Finally, judging (J) types preferred set patterns of times, orders and prayers, whereas perceiving (P) types preferred prayer that was flexible and open-ended.

Temperament may also be linked with different spiritualities (Michael and Norrisey, 1984; Richardson, 1996). There is currently limited empirical support for such correspondences, although Cook et al. (2025) and Francis et al. (2025) have found evidence in support of a link between Apollonian (NF) temperament and Augustinian spirituality amongst Anglican ordinands.

Prayer preferences may also relate to subclinical expressions of psychopathology. For example, different forms of narcissism have been linked with different kinds of prayer (Van Uden and Zondag, 2011; Zondag and Uden, 2014). Overt narcissism is associated with preferences for meditative and psychological prayer, whereas covert narcissism is associated with religious and petitionary prayer.

Prayer and Mental Health

Praying has been shown in research to be associated with a lower prevalence of depression, greater optimism, happiness, improved coping and better mental health (Robbins et al., 2008; Baesler and Ladd, 2009; Anderson and Nunnelley, 2016). Having someone pray with you can have a beneficial effect on both anxiety and depression (Boelens et al., 2009, 2012). Prayer has been shown to be associated with reduced craving amongst members of Alcoholics Anonymous (Galanter et al., 2017). Prayer may be beneficial for medical staff as well as for patients, helping in coping and remaining calm when working in a stressful environment (Cain, 2019; Achour et al., 2021).

Those who pray may have various expectations concerning the ways in which God may intervene in the world in response to their prayers. Leaving aside for a moment questions of divine intervention of a supernatural kind, there are many mechanisms by way of which prayer might be thought to be psychologically beneficial for those who pray (Breslin and Lewis, 2008).

Prayer may reduce experiential avoidance, the tendency to avoid unpleasant emotional states, which – in turn – is associated with psychopathology and poor outcomes (Lowe et al., 2022). The benefits of prayer may also be mediated by trust-based beliefs concerning when, where and how prayers are answered (Possel et al., 2014) or by 'disclosure to God', in which thoughts, experiences and feelings are shared with God in an interpersonal way (Winkeljohn Black et al., 2017).

The benefits of personal prayer are not invariable and may be dependent upon the image of God held in the mind of the person concerned. Images of an intimate relationship with a loving God are beneficial, but perceptions of God as impersonal or remote may be associated with a positive relationship between prayer and psychopathology (Bradshaw et al., 2008; Froese et al., 2024). Whilst much of the research has been undertaken on Christian samples, there is some evidence that benefits may vary for different kinds of prayer and for different faith traditions (Jeppsen et al., 2022).

Working with the Poloma and Pendleton typology, in a study of 296 Christian adults, Winkeljohn Black et al. (2015) found that colloquial and meditative prayer showed positive associations with mental health (as measured by the Profile of Mood States – Short Form), mediated by disclosure. Petitionary prayer showed a negative relationship with mental health and ritual prayer showed a positive relationship (but neither was associated with disclosure). The authors understand colloquial and meditative prayer as involving introspection and meaningful communication, whereas petitionary prayer is said to involve communication but not introspection. Ritual prayer, they somewhat prejudicially and questionably assert, 'does not have to require communication with God' (p.543).

In a study of anxiety, using her dimensional approach to measuring reasons for praying, Upenieks (2023) found that prayer efficacy, prayer for support and prayer for forgiveness (an aspect of devotional prayer) were all associated with higher anxiety. Praise of God (another aspect of devotional prayer) and prayer expectancy were associated with lower anxiety. However, in common with many other studies, the design of this one was cross-sectional and so it is not possible to infer causality. It may well be that anxious people are simply more likely to pray and that anxiety is thus the cause, rather than the effect, of prayer. The authors again acknowledge that images of God (not examined in this study) may influence relationships between prayer and mental health.

Coping Prayer

Prayer is probably the most widely used method of spiritual/religious coping worldwide. As such, depending upon the context and the person praying, it may function in a variety of beneficial ways.

In a study of US military veterans (Tait et al., 2016), a Prayer Functions Scale was used to study four different ways in which prayer is thought to help with coping: acceptance, calm and focus, assistance, and deferring/avoiding. Prayers for divine assistance, and for calm and focus, were associated with lower post-traumatic stress disorder (PTSD) symptomatology and less depression. Prayers asking God to intervene and resolve or remove the stressful situation (e.g., 'Pray for difficulties to be taken away') were associated with greater symptomatology of depression (but not PTSD). One might have imagined that the deferring/avoiding kind of prayer would be associated with reluctance to talk about experiences of trauma, but this was in fact not the case. The authors propose that prayer (of all types) is a kind of 'disclosure to God'. They caution that, whilst there might be potential clinical applications of their research, it would be necessary first to explore the nature of patients' God images before promoting prayer coping, lest negative forms of religious coping should inadvertently be encouraged.

Prayer may function in a variety of ways as a coping resource. In a qualitative study of 10 Roman Catholics who regularly used the rosary for prayer (Stöckigt et al., 2021), it was reported that prayer helped to manage stress, anxiety and sadness. Rosary prayer was described as facilitating acceptance, humility and devotion to God. In a study of 36 Christian subjects in the USA (Bade and Cook, 2008), prayer was found to support problem engagement (attempts to solve or remove the problem), emotion management and avoidance (distancing from the problem). A fourth function of prayer was identified in terms of cognitive reappraisal – a positive theological reframing of problems.

Different types of prayer may be mapped onto the wider research on religious coping. In a study of 336 Dutch and Flemish people (slightly less than half of whom identified as Christian), three types of prayer were identified: religious (focussed on relationship with God), petitionary (focussed on particular needs or problems) and meditative (understood as focussed on the self and/or the process of prayer itself) (Bänziger et al., 2008b). Religious prayer was found to be associated with Pargament's collaborative and deferring coping styles. Meditative prayer was associated with 'receptivity' (a religious coping style concerned more with acceptance than modification of life problems). Interestingly, petitionary prayer was not associated (as the authors had expected it would be) with a deferring style of religious coping.

The coping functions of prayer are related positively to post-traumatic growth (Harris et al., 2010). Post-traumatic growth is concerned with such things as relating to others, finding new possibilities in life, personal strength, spiritual growth and appreciation of life. The 'calm and focus' function of prayer (measured with the Prayer Functions Scale) is positively correlated with post-traumatic growth, at least for non-interpersonal trauma (e.g., natural disaster) amongst Christian subjects in the USA.

Prayer as Encounter

Prayer is commonly understood as an interpersonal encounter with a transcendent Other. Thus, for example, the Spanish mystic St Teresa of Avila (1515–1582) saw prayer in terms of friendship with God (Fernandez and Francis, 2022). Schjoedt et al. (2009), using fMRI to study a group of 20 Danish Christians, found that prayer activated areas of the brain usually employed in social cognition. It has been suggested that prayer in a scanner is not the same as 'normal' prayer (Ladd et al., 2015). However, I have prayed in an MRI scanner many times and would question this. Prayer takes many forms and is practised in many different contexts; it would not be expected to be exactly the same in all aspects in all times and in all places.

Ladd et al. (2012) have drawn attention to measurable differences in interpersonal communication with friends as compared with God. In a largely female group of psychology students, greater variety of language was reported in human–human interpersonal conversations than in prayer. Happiness and surprise were more commonly reported in human–human conversations, as compared with disgust, anger and fear in prayer. They suggest that this is because prayer has a stronger affective valence. Attachment patterns in human–human conversations and in prayer were found not to be correlated.

If prayer is understood as an encounter with a divine Other, then it is necessarily not only an encounter with (what we might call) the theological reality of that Other but also an encounter with projections of our own images of God formed in infancy (see Chapter 4). This is problematic not only because many people do not allow those images to develop with them into adulthood but also because such images easily become idolatrous representations which are substituted for the theological reality (Ulanov and Ulanov, 1985, pp.27–33). Self-images and God images have a complex interrelationship (MacKenna, 2002).

Attention

Simone Weil (1909–1943), the French philosopher and mystic, suggested that 'Absolutely unmixed attention is prayer' (Weil, 1952, p.106). For Weil, attention 'taken to its highest degree' can be considered prayer because it 'presupposes faith and love' (p.105). Many might argue that this is a big presupposition, but Weil argues that if we give our attention excessively to the wrong thing, for example a problem that we face, it is self-defeating. (This is not to say that we should not attend to our problems, only that the objects of our attention can sometimes be unhealthy, and that the form of our attending can be self-defeating.) On the other hand: 'If we turn our mind to the good, it is impossible that little by little the whole soul will not be attracted thereto in spite of itself' (p.106).

For Weil, 'attention' has a spiritual, contemplative quality which is not merely a psychological faculty (Delaruelle, 2003, p.20). In contrast, for Tanya Luhrmann (2020), an anthropologist and psychologist, it is a form of metacognition: 'The central act of praying is paying attention to inner experience – to thoughts, images, and the awareness of one's body – and treating those sensations as important in themselves rather than as distractions from the real business of living' (p.139). This metacognition is not a narcissistic or self-serving exercise. Rather, those who pray 'look back on their thoughts as if from outside and ask whether those thoughts are in accord with a world in which gods and spirits matter' (p.139). This process, as Luhrmann understands it, has benefits for emotional regulation, albeit that is not the primary motivation for engaging in it. In a psychological reformulation of Kierkegaard's assertion that prayer changes people, Luhrmann argues that 'Prayer changes people because prayer alters the way people attend to their own mental processes' (Luhrmann, 2020, p.139).

Theologically, it is not the psychological process – the metacognition – that is the essence of prayer. Rather, as St John of the Cross (1542–1591) suggested, the one who prays is ultimately called to 'Preserve a loving attentiveness to God with no desire to feel or understand any particular thing concerning him' (Kavanaugh and Rodriguez, 1991, p.92). This challenging call to radical attentiveness motivated by love is made possible by metacognitive processes, but it is not constituted by them. Prayer is a receptive, contemplative exercise in theological listening. Much of the scientific research reviewed earlier focusses on prayer in a utilitarian way which fails to recognise both the spiritual/contemplative and the metacognitive dimensions of prayer.

Whilst this core attentional focus of prayer is held in common by almost all faith traditions, it also reveals differences between them and within them. There is not space here to engage in a wide-ranging comparative religious study of prayer. However, it may be helpful to take one example. In Islam, proper intention (*niyya*) (Katz, 2013, pp.44–55) is central to understanding the nature of canonical prayer (*salat*). Salat, performed five times each day by observant Muslims, is concerned with reverence towards God and obedience to what God has commanded. Salat places emphasis on praying as part of a group (Al-Krenawi and Graham, 2000) and, even when Muslims do pray alone, the repetition and rituals characteristic of group prayer are integral to the prayers that are offered (Haeri, 2013). It is easy to fall into a trap of seeing niyya as a kind of interior psychological aspect of prayer, the spiritual inner correlate of the outward actions, but this is to misunderstand the nature of Islamic spirituality (Powers, 2004). Right intention (niyya) is not an interior aspect of an outward act but, rather, an integral part and parcel of prayer that gives proper attention to God. Prayer in Islam is, we might say, a thoroughly biopsychosocially integrated event.

Salat is not the only kind of prayer in Islam. *Du'a*, informal prayer, is concerned with making requests to God. Du'a raises interesting theological and psychological questions in relation to the attentional focus of prayer. Even assuming that requests made to God in prayer are not selfish and materialistic, they can still imply dissatisfaction with the way that God has ordered things. As Marion Holmes Katz puts it, there is 'a fine line between supplication and complaining' (Katz, 2013, p.34). On the other hand, the emotional sincerity of crying out to God from the depths of one's heart can be understood to draw one closer to God (as, for example, also happens in the Hebrew Psalms). The strong emphasis in Islam that the attentional focus of prayer is properly on God can thus create a psychological tension (between supplication and acceptance) for the one offering prayer in respect of their personal needs and concerns (Katz, 2013, pp.34–36).

By way of comparison, Sufism, a more interiorly focussed and mystical strand of Islam, prioritises a training of the inner senses (Luhrmann, 2020, p.73) and emphasises a third kind of prayer, remembrance of God (*dhikr*) (Brown, 2009, pp.199–202). Dhikr may take a variety of forms, including vocal or silent repetition of a confession of faith, or other religious words, attention to breathing, dancing, music or calligraphy (Aslan, 2011, pp.221–223). Whilst one might expect that Sufism would have even greater concerns about the problems inherent in du'a, in fact the opposite seems to be the case (Katz, 2013, pp.34–35).

Shamanic practices, such as those discussed by Olga Kharitidi (see Chapter 1), similarly give priority to inner experience (Noll, 1985), as do many strands of Christian and other forms of religious mysticism. Different traditions of prayer, with different theologies, give attention differently, and the psycho-theological tension between giving attention to God and attention to human needs is managed in various ways. However, not all religions are theistic, and Buddhism provides an interesting example of spiritual practice that does not give attention to God but nonetheless recognises that attentional focus is psychologically problematic.

Mindfulness

Mindfulness, a practice with its roots in Buddhism, has become an important spiritual intervention in mental health care (Mace, 2008). Mindfulness, like prayer, is integrally concerned with the giving of attention. Chris Mace (2008, p.4) suggests that 'to be mindful ... is to pay attention in a particular way'. This raises the question of exactly what that 'particular way' might be. He offers definitions from five different authors, each of whom emphasises something different. For example, for Kabat-Zinn, mindfulness is concerned with *'paying attention on purpose, in the present moment, and non-judgementally'* (Kabat-Zinn, 2020, p.xxxvii, original emphasis preserved). This definition emphasises intentionality, and the cognitive processes involved. However, for others, the emphasis variously falls on breadth of awareness, internal bodily processes such as breathing, or else on love and kindness (Mace, 2008, p.5). For the Buddhist monk Nyanaponika Thera (1901–1994), mindfulness is best understood as a form of 'bare attention', that is, awareness of things stripped of self-interest in such a way that we begin to see them differently (Gethin, 2011). Peter Tyler (2014), a Christian psychotherapist, has suggested that mindfulness is 'appropriate attention', raising the questions of what is appropriate and what it is that we attend to.

The widespread uptake of mindfulness as therapy has been made possible by the research evidence base that supports its impact on outcomes (Goldberg et al., 2018), and the relative ease of detaching it from its Buddhist roots. There is now agreement that mindfulness-based treatments are beneficial in relation to a range of mental health conditions, including depression, anxiety, stress and addiction (Zhang et al., 2021). However, to view it in these utilitarian terms is to wrench it from the Buddhist spiritual context within which it belongs. This has significant consequences. For example, an over-emphasis on mindfulness as non-judgemental risks losing sight of the Buddhist aim of addressing human greed, anger and delusion (the last of these terms being used in a particular Buddhist sense related to human ignorance/forgetfulness) (Gethin, 2011).

Dhyana (attention) plays an important part in Hinduism, Sikhism and Jainism, as well as in Buddhism (Singh, 2023). Mindfulness also has strong similarities to meditative and contemplative practices in Christianity, Judaism and Islam (Koenig, 2023). It is therefore not surprising that many Christians (Tyler, 2018) and Muslims (Aldbyani, 2024) find no conflict between their religious faith and the practice of mindfulness. Where potential concerns are identified, interestingly, these tend to be around the emphasis on mindfulness as non-judgemental (Hoover, 2018; Abdulkerim and Li, 2022), thus echoing exactly the same concerns that Buddhists have themselves. Further, there is evidence that mindfulness helps Christian mental health practitioners to integrate spirituality into their clinical work and to be more aware of the divine presence in their interactions with their patients (Trammel, 2017). Muslims who offer prayer (salat) regularly are more mindful in prayer, and experience better mental health, than those who do not pray regularly (Ijaz et al., 2017).

The word mindfulness is customarily employed as translation of the Pali word *sati* and/ or the Sanskrit word *smrti* (Gethin, 2011). The field of meaning of the original words of the

Buddhist texts is complex, also encompassing such things as remembrance and recollection. Tyler (2014) has suggested that a better translation might be 'heartfulness' or 'soulfulness'. He finds a close resonance with the writings on 'mental prayer' of the Spanish mystic Teresa of Avila. Tyler acknowledges an important theological distinction between the Christian prayer of recollection as practised by Teresa and the Buddhist practice of mindfulness. Teresa is focussed on a loving personal relationship with Jesus in prayer, something alien to Buddhism. However, he also points to the way in which both move attention away from intellectual, mental activity towards concerns of 'the heart'. Teresa's Spanish *oración mental* (mental prayer) might therefore better be translated as mindfulness than as mental prayer, if the latter implies something rational/intellectual rather than heartful.

This is not the place to elaborate further on the linguistic, theological and philosophical issues involved in comparisons of prayer and mindfulness. As psychiatrists, however, it is important that we observe that both are intimately involved with what we pay attention to, and how we pay attention, and that this in turn is closely connected with evidenced pathways to mental well-being and recovery. Prayer and mindfulness, if not exactly the same thing, are closely related to each other, and to the kinds of attention that a good clinician gives to his or her patients in person-centred care.

Paying Attention in Psychiatry

Good clinicians give careful attention to their patients. By this I mean not just attention to the diagnostic questions that patients raise for them, or to the scientific debates concerning evidenced-based treatments, but to the patient as a person. Attention is a core component of effective psychotherapy, and one which is too infrequently discussed (Speeth, 1982).

Marion Milner (1900–1998), a psychoanalyst, wrote her influential study *On Not Being Able to Paint* well before mindfulness had become an important topic of conversation in mental health care in the Western world (Milner, 1950). In it, she distinguishes between two kinds of attention – the narrowly focussed attention of which scientific objectivity is a leading example, and a broader, unfocussed attention that apprehends 'the unique reality of a person as of a picture' (p.99). The former, narrower kind of attention she found was non-embracing, unable by its very nature to 'encompass a wholeness' (p.125). She came to realise that 'scientific objectivity was only a partial aspect of one's relation to the world, and that both ways of looking were sterile without each other. In fact, one had to stand apart in order once more to come together again in a restored wholeness of perception' (p.99). I think that this broader, unfocussed, attention – which apprehends the 'pictures' of people as persons – is closely aligned to mindfulness and prayer. When I was running a spirituality group for patients in a community service for people with drinking problems, one of my patients discovered something of this sort quite unexpectedly:

> He had heard that fossil sharks' teeth could often be found on a local beach when the tide receded beyond a certain point. Some of these teeth appeared intact, others set in rocks or surrounded by pebbles, stone and chalk. He was fascinated by the indeterminable age of these teeth, their origins and symbolism. Thus, on one particular day, he set out with his daughter, in her early twenties, with whom he had a close relationship, to work methodically up and down the beach, a set distance apart, silent so as to concentrate and speaking only to announce a find. After some time, he realized that when they stuck to this method they rarely, if ever, struck lucky. However – and this was not conscious but noted in hindsight – when their silent searching was fruitless and they started talking, walking together and taking in all their

surroundings, they frequently 'stumbled upon' a tooth or two. Buoyed by this, they became aware that they were deviating from their set plan and moved back into position, confident of success as, after all, if the teeth could be stumbled across, think how many could be found with a little organization! And so the cycle repeated. Musing upon this in the group, the [patient] was struck by the beauty of this apparent unconscious order that manifest [sic] when consciousness was bypassed. But he was also frustrated by the paradoxical impossibility of such a process, in that he felt unable to accept that this is how such things worked, but rather strove to understand and master. (Jackson and Cook, 2005, pp.379–380)

Iain McGilchrist (2011) similarly recognises two kinds of attention, based upon the different ways in which the two cerebral hemispheres function. He points out that we need both kinds of attention, but that the way in which we use them determines the way in which we see the world: 'Attention is reciprocally related to what exists: it's not just that we attend differently depending on what we find, but that what we find depends on the kind of attention we pay' (p.1068). The left hemisphere kind of attention, the narrowly focussing one that isolates, fragments, classifies and manages the world around us, providing us with certainty about things, does not on its own foster the practice of good medicine. Rather, the right hemisphere kind of attention, the kind that apprehends the whole human being amidst a network of relationships, accepting uncertainty and flux (and thus able to accommodate religious ways of seeing the world (McGilchrist, 2019)), is needed in order for us to see people in all their meaningful complexity: 'Medicine is not about bodies, brains, or minds, but about human beings, their lives and experience. If practised attentively, it will lead to lesser, rather than greater, certainty about what on earth those bodies, brains, and minds might really be like' (McGilchrist, 2011, p.1069).

As clinicians, psychiatrists may not abandon the narrower kind of attentiveness without failing in their responsibility to be good scientists. They may not abandon the broader, non-embracing form of attention without failing in their obligations to person-centred care. This latter, I would argue, is at the spiritual heart of good psychiatric practice. However, as my patient vividly articulated, this can be very frustrating as it requires a certain amount of giving up of a 'left hemisphere' desire to control and master.

Adverse Effects

Prayer is affirmed as a beneficial spiritual practice by almost all faith traditions, but it also has its dark side. As Ashley Cocksworth (2023) has argued, prayer can become 'dehumanising, destructive, dangerous and damaging – more means of sin than means of grace' (p.12). Prayer becomes implicated in spiritual abuse, as in conversion therapies, and in patriarchal, political and colonial structures of power. It is all too easy to ask for the wrong things in prayer, so that prayer becomes shaped by unconscious biases, an expression of narcissistic and potentially dangerous and unexamined desires.

Prayer 'utterances' (public statements that one is praying about something) can function as 'aligning actions', associating the one praying with particular social norms and values, rather than primary concerns, so as to justify questionable and potentially problematic courses of action (Sharp, 2012). Prayer, as illustrated by Jenny's experiences in Chapter 1, can become entangled with psychopathology, for example in the religious rituals associated with some forms of OCD (Bonchek and Greenberg, 2009; Rahman et al., 2021b).

Mindfulness practice, although it fares well in comparison with other psychological treatments (Britton et al., 2021) and waiting list controls (Hirshberg et al., 2022), is probably also not completely harmless. It may be transiently anxiogenic (Aizik-Reebs et al., 2021) and, for some, associated with a deterioration of symptoms (Baer et al., 2021). Childhood trauma and symptoms of PTSD when treated with mindfulness-based interventions may have worse outcomes (Canby et al., 2025).

Praying with Patients

Many years ago, I heard it said that a Christian doctor is one who prays for his/her patients. I have reflected since that it depends very much on what you mean by 'prays for'. I have certainly always aspired to give careful and respectful attention to my patients, and (as discussed earlier) this is a kind of prayer. There is also a Christian tradition, dating back to St Benedict (480–547), that work is a form of prayer (Wirzba, 2006). My becoming a doctor was a prayer, my clinical work is prayer, and prayer is not something that is separate from the rest of my life. I have increasingly often asked God to bring healing to my patients, and have prayerfully remembered them after my clinics, but prayer is not just about words.

It is important to distinguish between praying for and praying with. A third category might be praying alongside (Ali, 2015). Each of these will have its own psychological and spiritual implications for clinical practice. Practitioners may be more aware of the potential dangers of praying with patients, and patients more aware of the potential benefits (Van Nieuw Amerongen-Meeuse et al., 2020).

In correspondence in *Psychiatric Bulletin* following publication of an editorial by Professor Harold Koenig (2008b), praying with patients became a particular focus of debate and controversy (see Chapter 8). Subsequently, Professor Rob Poole and I engaged in a published debate on the topic in the *British Journal of Psychiatry* (Poole and Cook, 2011). The motion for the debate was framed in the negative – 'Praying with a patient constitutes a breach of professional boundaries in psychiatric practice' (Poole and Cook, 2011, p.94) – and so Professor Poole went first in the debate in proposing the motion. I have often wondered what it would have been like if it had been the other way around. Why is it that the starting point for the debate should presume that prayer is the wrong thing to be doing with patients, rather than the right thing? In opening a positively framed motion I would have liked to begin with explorations of exactly what prayer with a patient is, and I would have found it difficult to define, precisely because prayer cannot be separated out from the rest of Christian life. (I write as a Christian, but I imagine that my Jewish, Muslim and other colleagues may have similar concerns.)

Praying with a patient is – at one level – something I cannot avoid doing as a Christian, simply by virtue of being a Christian doctor. Of course I realise that this is not what Professor Poole had in mind, but the debate thus started with his presuppositions rather than mine. Within the debate, we did explore the question of the nature of prayer – and Professor Poole was not impressed by my explanation. He did, however, clarify that 'There can be no objection to prayer that occurs implicitly or subliminally, any more than there can be an objection to implicit or unstated sexual attraction. It is when prayer is explicit and acted on within the relationship that a problem arises, just like sexual activity' (Poole and Cook, 2011, p.96). The comparison with sexual behaviour is interesting. Again, the argument presumes the negative: prayer in clinical practice is wrong, just as sex in clinical practice is wrong, and both are concerned with professional boundary breaking. I will return to the important question of boundary breaking in Chapter 8 but, for now, I want to explore the positive dimensions of 'praying with', which I still feel were rather sidelined in the *BJPsych* debate.

Sex is not wrong per se, but only when abused, especially in the context of a power differential such as that provided by professional medical practice. Similarly, prayer is not wrong per se, but only when abused. Unlike sex, prayer with others is widely, voluntarily and appropriately practised in public places around the world. The historical, cultural and geographical presumptions have much more been that praying with others is a good thing to do. Prayer, ideally, transcends boundaries rather than creating them. It does this only when it is non-coercive.

As explored earlier in this chapter, the psychological and the spiritual elements of prayer cannot be disentangled; they are inseparable. Psychology and theology each have their own contributions to make in exploring the nature of prayer, but prayer will always be at once a spiritual and a psychological endeavour. For religious people worldwide it is one of the most pervasive and powerful psychological realities that they experience daily. For psychiatrists, psychologists or psychotherapists to dismiss, neglect or proscribe this in relation to clinical practice is a curious form of anti-religious secular bias and a failure to attend to an aspect of life which can have potentially powerful positive or negative influences upon mental health outcomes.

Having said all of this, my praying with patients has almost always been of the silent and implicit kind. I can only remember one particular occasion when it was explicit and acted upon in the clinical context. Nothing dramatic happened. My patient (let's call her Susan) was suffering from depression and was receiving a prescription from me for antidepressant medication. She had asked to see me because she was a Christian and wanted to see a Christian psychiatrist. I'm sure that I would have said then, as I have so often since to others, that she needed a 'good' psychiatrist, not necessarily a Christian one. However, on this occasion I was the responsible clinician, and (unusually) my identity as a Christian was known to my patient. She asked me if I would pray with her at the end of one of our outpatient encounters, and I agreed.

Some psychiatrists may have concerns that my praying with Susan had psychological consequences, and I accept that it altered my relationship with her. For a few moments of prayer, we were two Christians praying together that God would bring one of us healing. I was no longer the source of healing towards which Susan looked. I could easily have abused this opportunity to pray if I had consciously or subconsciously wanted to, but rather I kept my prayer short and asked simply for that which all doctors and patients seek – that there may be healing. It is my belief that this strengthened the therapeutic alliance and contextualised the clinical encounter within a transcendent frame of reference which was both psychologically and spiritually helpful for Susan.

Had I refused to pray with Susan, I think that I would undoubtedly have damaged the therapeutic relationship. Depending upon how clumsily or sensitively I had managed my refusal, I might have come across as uncaring, aloof or arrogant. I would certainly have damaged Susan's trust in my concern for her and in her need to be understood as a whole person, body, mind and spirit. Given her depressive illness, this may well have reinforced her negative cognitions, damaged her already fragile sense of self-worth and undermined the positive potential for her to use spiritual/religious coping as a valuable resource to aid in her recovery.

Praying with Susan also had a positive effect on me. It was – and is – a reminder that, whilst I do what I can, there is so much in clinical practice that is beyond my understanding and which I cannot change. It is helpful, as a clinician, to have the humility to acknowledge that I am not God, and that I share with my patients a precarious existence on a small planet orbiting a small star amidst a vast universe. Ultimately, it is God who brings healing, not me. All psychiatrists have worldviews which may potentially influence their clinical practice. It is incumbent upon all clinicians to reflect on how these worldviews influence their clinical practice, whether for good or ill.

My prayer with Susan was very much the exception in my clinical practice. Much more often, my prayers for my patients have been silent ones.

Silence

My understanding of the nature of prayer changed profoundly when my wife died (see Chapter 2). I don't think that I realised this at the time, but it is more obvious now looking back with the perspective of four decades. It made me more ready to sit with the silences of others, and (eventually) to find that silence was often a more effective prayer than could be offered in words. It made me more aware of the gulf between the desires that I express verbally in prayer and what God may desire for me. Too often, our bids to fill silences with words (whether in prayer or in clinical practice) are an uneasy attempt to repress our own anxiety, and to avoid sharing in the suffering of others. Writing of his conversation with a victim of horrific violence at the hands of rebels, during the civil war in Sierra Leone, the anthropologist Michael Jackson suggests that loquacity 'risks doing violence to the very experiences it struggles to make sense of'. He continues:

> This is why our language must be measured and tempered, rather than used to fill silences, or speak that which the sufferer cannot speak. And this is why we should learn the value of silence, seeing it not as a sign of indifference or resignation, but of respect ... Silence is sometimes the only way we can honour the ineffability and privacy of certain experiences.
>
> Such silence may be, as in Africa, a way of healing and reconciliation, and not a way of evading or repressing an issue. (Jackson, 2004, p.56)

Silence is not just the absence of noise. In fact, there is evidence to suggest that silence is actively perceived, rather than just being a failure to hear (Goh et al., 2023). It is thus something that may be actively attended to, as in various spiritual practices, including contemplative prayer. Alexander Ryrie, an Episcopalian priest, writes in *The Prayer of Silence*: 'Underlying all our prayer there is silence. It is the basis of our relationship with God; through it we relate to God and God relates to us. Silence is a deep and incomprehensible mystery. It is not simply an absence of noise, but something real and positive' (Ryrie, 2012, p.27).

There are many kinds of silence, notably, for our present purpose, inner silences (concerned with the kind of inner chatter that mindfulness seeks to address) and external silences, including those that emerge in clinical practice. The latter have been defined as 'moments within the therapy session in which dialogue is halted' (Levitt and Morrill, 2023, p.321). This hardly does justice to their psychological significance. For Freud, silences that emerged in the course of therapy were interpreted in a largely negative manner as defensive or hostile. However, the interplay between speech and silence is more complex than this; silence may be productive and communicative, and an abundance of words may be self-protective or aggressive. Speech and silence may be understood as oppositional, but in need of each other. A Jungian perspective might therefore rather seek to find the transcendent function that emerges from their union (or *coniunctio*, to employ the Jungian terminology), rather than imposing one at the expense of the other (Bravesmith, 2012).

Silence arises within a biopsychosocial matrix. There is evidence to suggest that inner silence and outer silence have different effects on the autonomic nervous system, with the latter producing heightened alertness and the former reducing sympathetic activity and stress (Donelli et al., 2023). The depth of mental silence achieved during Sahaja yoga meditation correlates with grey matter volumes in the medial prefrontal cortex, a brain region known to be important for top-down processes such as emotional regulation (Hernandez et al., 2018). Silence training, in long-term Vipassana meditators, is associated with decoupling of brain language networks from the default mode network and an inverse correlation with activity of the dorsal attention network (Tripathi et al., 2024). Whilst these cross-sectional studies cannot demonstrate causality, they do suggest that meditation practice improves ability to manage internal and external distractions.

A rather different kind of silence, mnemonic silence – a refusal or failure to remember in the course of social discourse – can have differential impact on speaker and listener, and, depending upon the type of silence, can aid (or in some cases impair) forgetting (Stone et al., 2012). On the other hand, as with the commonly observed two minutes' silence on Remembrance Day, silence may provide a way of remembering. In each case, it has psychological and social significance. It is a way of giving attention to things, both those that are remembered and – sometimes paradoxically – those that are not.

Silence has received particular attention in the practice of psychotherapy (Levitt and Morrill, 2023). Silence as a psychotherapeutic intervention can be a way of communicating empathy, facilitating reflection or expression of feelings, putting the onus on the patient to initiate/speak, or thinking about what to say next (Ladany et al., 2006). It needs to be contained within the safe boundaries of a good therapeutic relationship and is best avoided in certain situations (e.g., when the patient is psychotic, angry or anxious) (Ladany et al., 2006). If used inappropriately, silence can convey distance, lack of interest or disengagement, and can damage the therapeutic alliance or make the patient feel unsafe (Lane et al., 2002). On the other hand, compassionate silences can emerge during clinical practice, in which healing can be facilitated. These are made possible by 'the clinician who has developed mental capacities of stable attention, emotional balance, along with prosocial mental qualities, such as naturally arising empathy and compassion' (Back et al., 2009 , p.1114). These qualities are mindful, but they also derive from contemplative practices which may be helpful for therapists (Rajski, 2003), as well as for their patients.

Silence has important linguistic and spiritual significance. Ivan Illich has suggested that 'The learning of a language is more the learning of its silences than its sounds ... The learning of the grammar of silence is an art much more difficult to learn than the grammar of sounds' (Illich, 1973, p.41). He suggests a classification of silences (which he acknowledges is not exhaustive), including a silence before words (a silence of listening), the silence of syntony and a silence beyond words. Each has its positive and negative forms, which he understands in accordance with his Christian tradition, but he sees them culminating in a particular form of silence beyond words – that of the mystery of death. The various shapes of silence might be somewhat differently conceived in different faith traditions but, I would suggest, this general pattern draws attention to a dynamic of silence which is beyond any particular faith tradition.

The intention here is not to impose prayer or silence on all psychiatrists but, rather, to invite reflection on the ways in which silence may draw together psychiatrists and patients from diverse backgrounds and beliefs, whether or not prayer might be a part of their vocabulary. Silence plays an important part in interfaith dialogue (Aguilar, 2017). Silence occupies an important place in palliative care, especially in the context of discussing spiritual or existential concerns (Bassett et al., 2018). I see no reason why it should not occupy a similar place in psychiatry.

It has been a long tradition within the Spirituality and Psychiatry Special Interest Group (SPSIG) that we begin executive meetings, and sometimes other events, with a short period of silence. I imagine that some members of the group are mindful but not prayerful; others may be prayerful but not mindful; and probably many are both. Silence operates in a unique way as a language of spirituality that enables attention to be given to the ineffable across boundaries of theology, culture or faith (Butler and Butler, 1996, pp.76–90; Kenny, 2021).

Attentive Psychiatry

Prayer, mindfulness and silence are deeply entangled. Each has a research evidence base to support the contention that it has an important part to play in patient-centred clinical practice. Ultimately, the reason for considering such things is not a utilitarian focus on outcomes (important though that may be) so much as an understanding of the need to pay careful and compassionate attention, to the present moment, to the human condition and to the theological and spiritual context within which patients understand themselves and their distress. They do also have an impact on outcomes, but they more importantly stretch our thinking about what outcomes we are really looking for.

Prayer, mindfulness and silence offer different ways in which psychiatrists and, more importantly, patients may keep spirituality in mind when planning treatment. In a sense, treatment planning in psychiatry is a particular kind of prayer (broadly conceived), a mindful attentiveness to what our patients truly desire. Such attentiveness, whatever the theologies (or atheologies) of clinician and patient, both acknowledges and affirms the spirituality inherent in the biopsychosocial matrix with which psychiatry is centrally concerned. As I wrote elsewhere (in relation to Christian spirituality, but I think the point is equally applicable to the spiritualities of other traditions): 'We need to get better at seeing a daily dose of medication as a prayer for healing (where the act of taking medication becomes prayerful), and a prayer offered from a place of emotional darkness as an important psycho-spiritual therapy' (Cook et al., 2023, p.133).

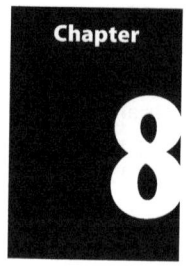

Psychiatrists and Spirituality

It is not necessary to have experienced mental illness to be a good psychiatrist, but it is necessary to be able to reflect on experiences of being human. Some refer to patients as 'experts by experience', but experience does not necessarily bring with it the ability to reflect wisely. It is this capacity for self-reflection on one's own inner life and experiences which, I would suggest, is an essential aspect of being a good psychiatrist. It helps us to care well for others whose experiences of illness have been a cause of inner turmoil and distress for them. Empathy, if not sympathy, is an important part of good professional practice.

Psychoanalysts have, as a core requirement of training, an expectation of undergoing their own analysis as a basis for the personal formation that makes a good analytic therapist. In the same way, given the entanglements of psychiatry with spirituality discussed earlier in this book, it might be argued that the good psychiatrist needs, at least, to be able to reflect on their own spiritual perspectives and the ways in which these might variously aid or hinder a good therapeutic relationship with patients. I am, of course, including here those perspectives that might be labelled as agnostic, atheist or 'neither spiritual nor religious', as well as those that are explicitly theological or religious. However, given the entanglements, such processes of spiritual formation and professional development may potentially be problematic. In particular, they raise serious concerns around professional practice and boundaries.

The concept of secularisation might have led some to suppose that religion no longer has a part to play in public life, and that the delivery of healthcare should necessarily be a secular and not a religious matter (unless, perhaps, sometimes delivered privately by religious organisations to those who wish to receive healthcare within such a context). However, the secularisation theory has major weaknesses (Martin, 2005), and religion is now seen to play a prominent part in public life, both in plural societies such as India or parts of the UK, and in countries where religion and politics are more or less inseparable, such as many nations in the Middle East or parts of the USA. Secularism is itself a plurality, expressing itself differently in different times and places, and some have suggested that we have now entered a post-secular age (Damberg Nissen et al., 2018). Recent research shows that the UK is one of the least religious countries in the world (Evans, 2024). We have a skewed perspective on the importance of religion worldwide, and a blindness to its importance for those communities within our own nation in which it occupies a central place in daily life. It might be argued that we have a prejudice against the global majority perspective on spirituality and religion.

On the other hand, the concept of religion has come under scrutiny in recent years, and may be understood as a product of colonial imperialism (Bergunder, 2014) which has a questionable place in a decolonised curriculum and a post-colonial world. Spirituality, for many, has become more important than religion, such as for those whose personal identity might be understood more as spiritual but not religious (SBNR) (Mercadante, 2014). Even for those who are 'religious' in a technical sense, there may be serious questions about religious institutions, and their desire may be to focus more on personal spirituality. For others, personal identity as either spiritual or religious is rejected completely and alternative worldviews are adopted, perhaps focussing on similar concerns but using a different vocabulary, such as relationality or meaning and purpose in life.

In the latter part of the twentieth century, a variety of factors converged to generate both interest and concern in relation to spirituality and religion in psychiatry (Cook, 2020b). On the one hand, research publications generated a growing evidence base suggesting that spirituality/religion might actually be good for mental health in various ways. On the other hand, concerns arose – notably in the USA – around ways in which the spirituality/religion of the psychiatrist might sometimes adversely affect clinical practice (Galanter et al., 1991). At the same time, the public debate, within the profession and more widely, began to engage with the topic in a new way, breaking the relative silence that had prevailed since the era of Freud and Jung.

In this context, over several decades, there have been a variety of policy initiatives in different countries, and development of guidelines for good practice. This debate has been generated by those who have concerns about adverse ways in which spirituality/religion may impact upon clinical practice as much as, or more than, those who advocate for addressing spirituality/religion in their clinical work. Doubtless some psychiatrists are indifferent or wonder what the fuss is all about. However, the debate has included the whole profession, and valuable contributions have been made by antagonists as much as by protagonists.

At the same time, there have been gatherings of national and international groups of psychiatrists who come together to discuss their shared interests as protagonists of the giving of a greater profile to spirituality/religion in clinical practice. These gatherings, both virtual and face to face, address not only the concerns of patients but also the spiritual challenges of being a psychiatrist. Because such groups almost always include a diversity of spiritual and religious perspectives, they might be understood as more or less uneasy coalitions, or as places in which to have safe conversation over differences, as much as groups of like-minded individuals.

The present chapter will consider some of the key themes arising from these debates, as well as examples of the guidelines that have emerged in different contexts. The implications for patient-centred practice will be explored, drawing on examples of some of the clinical scenarios that generate the debates and raise questions about the nature of good practice.

Spirituality as 'Special Interest'

A Committee on Relations between Psychiatry and Religion was authorised by the American Psychiatric Association (APA) as early as 1956. The present APA Caucus on Spirituality, Religion and Psychiatry, convened in 2012, continues the work of this group (Cook, 2022e, p.8). In the UK, through the 1990s, high-profile lectures addressing spirituality/religion were given to the Royal College of Psychiatrists by successive presidents of the College, by the Archbishop of Canterbury and by the College's patron, HRH The Prince of Wales (now King Charles III) (Cook, 2020b). In 1999, a Spirituality and Psychiatry Special Interest Group (SPSIG) was established within the RCPsych, with the intention to 'facilitate the exchange of ideas on a wide range of topics, including the significance of the major religions which influence the values and beliefs of the society in which we live, also taking into account the spiritual aspirations of individuals who do not identify with any one particular faith and those who hold that spirituality is independent of religion' (Shooter, 1999). This group has subsequently flourished and, at the time of writing, its membership comprises approximately one-quarter of the total College membership.

Similar national groups – variously named – now exist in at least seven other countries. In 2003, a Section on Religion, Spirituality and Psychiatry was established within the World Psychiatric Association (WPA). These groups variously exist to influence clinical practice, foster research and improve education on spirituality/religion in relation to psychiatry.

Professional Debate

This wave of interest in spirituality and religion has not been without controversy and the question arises as to whether spirituality/religion are properly a 'special interest' for some within psychiatry, or actually more fundamental and essential aspects of clinical practice and research which should be the concern of all members of the profession. Some might wish to propose an opposite, and even more radical, question, namely, whether spirituality/religion should have any place in psychiatry at all – although the exact framing of that question might be nuanced in various ways. Clearly, the topic cannot realistically be completely proscribed, given that many patients may want to bring it up in the consulting room, and it is difficult to see why they should not be allowed to do so. The question is therefore – more exactly – about where precisely the boundaries should be drawn.

An illustrative example arises in relation to an editorial published in *Psychiatric Bulletin* in 2008 under the title 'Religion and Mental Health: What Should Psychiatrists Do?'. Written by Harold Koenig (2008b), as a leading researcher in the field and a clinical psychiatrist, this short piece essentially affirmed the importance of addressing spirituality/religion in clinical practice – just as many others had done previously. However, it generated a fierce controversy, particularly in relation to whether or not Professor Koenig's proposals represented a breaching of professional boundaries (Poole et al., 2008). Why was this?

Koenig's editorial began with a brief review of psychiatrists' religious beliefs, attitudes and practices, drawing attention to issues of psychiatrists' personal non-belief (encountered more frequently than amongst patients), and a mixed picture of understanding the relationship between religion/mental illness. As Professor Poole and his colleagues pointed out in correspondence, there is good news here as well as bad: 'religion can be both helpful and problematic to service users' (Poole et al., 2008, p.356). However, Poole also, surprisingly, stated that since 1978 neither he nor any of his seven co-authors had ever encountered denigration or attack of religion by psychiatrists. Apart from my own experience that this does happen, and complaints that I have received from various patients about their psychiatrists' lack of religious sensitivity, there is well-known published research outlining concerns of patients about such problems (Macmin and Foskett, 2004).

After this preamble, Koenig focussed on 'taking a spiritual history, supporting healthy religious beliefs, challenging unhealthy beliefs, praying with patients (in highly selected cases) and consultation with, referral to, or joint therapy with trained clergy' (Koenig, 2008b, p.201). In the flurry of ensuing correspondence, a number of issues proved highly controversial including, notably: the potential intrusiveness of the spiritual history; the difficulties of distinguishing between those religious beliefs that should be supported and those that should be challenged; and the suggestion that the psychiatrist might sometimes pray with a patient. In each case, the concern was expressed that such recommendations could lead to breaches of professional boundaries. These boundaries (about which I have written in more detail elsewhere – Cook, 2013a, 2020b) include, notably: the boundary of specialist expertise; the boundary between the secular and the spiritual/religious; and the boundary between personal and professional life and values. Taking these in turn, it is first certainly clear that many psychiatrists do not feel adequately trained to address issues of spirituality/religion arising in clinical practice. The obvious response to this would be to improve training. Just as clergy need to better understand mental health as it relates to their primary role of spiritual care, so psychiatrists need to better understand spirituality/religion in relation to their primary role of mental health care. Given that the two domains are entangled, as argued throughout this book, the realistic solution is not so much to try to disentangle them (which – I have been arguing – is an impossible task) but, rather, to understand the nature of the entanglement better and to work collaboratively (as Koenig argued we should) with chaplains, clergy and faith leaders.

Critics are quite right to point out that psychiatrists are not specialists in spirituality/religion. In fact, Koenig has elsewhere similarly argued that it is mental health chaplains who are the true specialists in this area (Koenig, 2013). The differences here seem (at least to me) to be more apparent than real. In patient-centred practice, the patient will always know more than the psychiatrist or the chaplain about their beliefs, values and worldview. The clinical task is to understand that patient-centred perspective as fully as possible, and to ensure that spiritual history taking is both relevant and affirmingly curious, not intrusive. Where a patient identifies with atheism or agnosticism, then this is just as important to understand as it would be if they were strongly religious or SBNR.

The second boundary, the boundary between the secular and the spiritual/religious, is, in fact, a part of the problem as far as many patients are concerned. That which is secular is not perceived as neutral; it is strongly biased against understandings of the transcendent (Cook et al., 2011). If psychiatry is in a quest for 'neutral' clinical space in which to operate, secularity is no better than religious space, unless of course you happen to be atheist or agnostic. In any case, all clinicians are human beings with their own beliefs about spirituality/religion, their own unconscious biases, and their own social and cultural contexts. As such, any 'secular' space can never be completely neutral, unless the spirituality/religion/(non-)beliefs of the psychiatrist entering it are somehow acknowledged, reflected upon and taken into account in clinical practice. If this is done properly, whether by atheists and agnostics or by those who are spiritual/religious, these beliefs can be an asset rather than a liability.

The problem, then, is not that psychiatrists are not experts on spirituality/religion, or that spirituality/religion are intruding upon 'safe' secular space (which is not actually safe at all for most patients), but rather that the psychiatrist has to be aware of, reflect upon and manage effectively the boundary between the professional and the personal in relation to spirituality/religion in patient-centred care. That this will sometimes be complicated, and even difficult, is not contested here. Patients will sometimes present problems relating to what we might call 'pathological' spirituality (Crowley and Jenkinson, 2022). In fact, there are a variety of criteria by way of which such mentally unhealthy cults and sects might be identified, and there is a body of literature relating to the most effective clinical responses to bring to bear in working with such patients. Similarly, psychiatrists may sometimes face their own challenges in reconciling their personal beliefs with the requirements of professional practice. This is exactly why groups such as the SPSIG and the APA Caucus are required, so as to create reflective space within which psychiatrists may safely explore such issues with their peers.

The problem, ultimately, is that God has no boundaries. Writing in reference to Christian meditation (but I daresay this could be true in most other theistic traditions too), Thomas Merton says: 'The infinite God has no boundaries and our minds cannot set limits to him or to his love. His presence is then "grasped" in the general awareness of loving faith, it is "realized" without being scientifically and precisely known' (Merton, 1969, p.109). Theologically, this is a matter of God's omnipresence (at least according to the Abrahamic faiths, but to a greater or lesser extent in other traditions too). Psychologically, it is a matter of what theist clinicians and patients inevitably bring into any situation. They cannot leave their beliefs about God outside the consulting room, as though these were optional accessories; rather, the thought of God is inevitably a part of every conversation, whether articulated or not. Thus, as inscribed over the door to Jung's home, 'Vocatus atque non vocatus Deus aderit' – 'Bidden or not, God is present'.[1]

Boundary-Breaking

Boundaries conceived of in an abstract way are one thing. Boundaries in actual clinical practice are quite another. The specifics of any particular case involve multiple variables of clinical history, cultural context, psychopathology, personality, family dynamics, therapeutic relationships and so much more. All of this assembles itself in human minds – at least for most of us – in the shape of narrative. Within these stories that we tell about ourselves, our patients and one another, there is scope for ethical principles to emerge in a bottom-up way, based on situational factors as much (or perhaps more) than the top-down systems of thinking that emerge from theology or philosophy.

In order to study how boundaries are understood by psychiatrists in practice, a group of four researchers developed a series of clinical vignettes, based upon actual cases (but suitably anonymised), as a tool for exploring attitudes to boundaries and boundary violations (Poole et al., 2024). The four researchers, amongst whom I was one, came from different personal perspectives: two Christians and two atheists; two psychiatrists, one theological ethicist and one social scientist. A part of the study (currently unpublished) concerned our own evaluation of the vignettes as researchers, but three of the vignettes were also used as a tool for discussion amongst 80 mental health professionals (most of whom were psychiatrists). The researchers then evaluated the responses of these clinicians, to determine whether or not each of the vignettes was assessed as a possible boundary violation, an actual boundary violation or no boundary violation.

The interesting finding of this research was that there was heterogeneity of opinion concerning boundary violations. Equivocation was common, pragmatic concerns came to the fore (rather than theological or philosophical arguments) and – even where there was agreement, in that all agreed that proselytising in clinical practice should not be allowed – there was lack of consensus about exactly what constituted proselytising. Outcomes featured as important in the thinking of our research subjects, but this became complicated in one particular case where the end (a good outcome) was not seen by all participants as justifying the means (a psychotherapeutic conversation about perceived spiritual realities).

---

[1] This quote is often attributed to Jung but is earlier attributable to the Dutch humanist Desiderius Erasmus (1469–1536). It is said that it originally derived from a Delphic oracle.

The three vignettes that were employed in this study were chosen from a larger bank of vignettes as having been particularly controversial. One of these concerned a junior psychiatrist seen to be reading a Bible with one of his patients. Relatively few participants (n=8) felt that there was definitely no boundary violation in this case, and the largest group (n=28) felt that there was a possible boundary violation, with most wanting more information about the circumstances surrounding the episode. However, a substantial number (n=19) seemed to feel that there was no need for further information in order to be clear that, for example, this behaviour was outside the role of a doctor and likely to cause disparity and exclusion within the wider group of patients on the ward.

A second vignette concerned a patient on a medical ward who was refusing to eat and drink, on the grounds that – as she understood it – she found a message in the Bible concerning purity and living on the Holy Spirit alone. After discussion with her priest and family, her Bible was taken away from her, and some research participants considered this to be a violation of her civil liberties. However, most (n=36) participants considered that there was no boundary violation in this case. Only a few participants (n=5) were certain that this case represented a boundary violation, and they were divided between those who were concerned about the removal of the Bible, and those who had concerns about the involvement of a priest.

The third of the three vignettes was the most controversial. A patient bereaved by suicide said that she was 'not feeling herself'. Invited by the psychiatrist to reflect on whether or not she was feeling like someone else, she entered into an imagined dialogue with the deceased friend and found herself giving voice to the deceased friend's regrets. The vignette ends with the spirit of the deceased friend (as represented by the patient) being ready to 'move on' and being invited to look to 'the light' and then leaving. For the largest group of research participants (n=32), this was seen to be a definite boundary violation. For some, the psychiatrist had provided a 'safe place' in which to explore an emotionally difficult loss, and the good outcome justified the therapeutic approach. For others, the psychiatrist had colluded with delusional conversation concerning 'a spirit'.

The important conclusions from this published research were concerning the use of the method (discussions concerning complex case vignettes) as a tool to explore boundaries, and the heterogeneity of views concerning exactly what the proper boundaries are. Whilst it is quite legitimate for clinicians to have different views on these matters, it does raise significant questions about what good practice looks like where we do not agree and where ethical principles are much more situationally specific than they are based upon agreed rules which can be clearly articulated and applied generally. It is also concerning that a patient's perfectly normal (for many) views about spiritual survival after death can be described by a psychiatrist as 'delusions'. Beliefs that may be completely normative for a patient (in the third vignette) can easily be seen by a psychiatrist as evidence of psychopathology. Similarly, in the first vignette, professional behaviour that may be appreciated by a patient (and may even have been invited by the patient) can be assumed to be unprofessional solely because it involves a religious object (a Bible).

Is it possible, given these situational specifics and the variety of professional opinions concerning them, to offer any general guidance as to what might constitute good psychiatric practice in relation to spirituality and religion? Judging by the number of attempts internationally to develop guidelines, one must assume that many psychiatrists believe that it is.

Guidelines

In 1991, the Committee on Religion and Psychiatry of the APA published *Guidelines Regarding Possible Conflict between Psychiatrists' Religious Commitments and Psychiatric Practice* (Committee on Religion and Psychiatry, 1990). An appendix to the Guidelines gave four examples of 'the kinds of problems that may arise when strong beliefs are interjected into a clinical practice'. These examples were one instance of a psychiatrist who considered his patient's sexual orientation to be sinful; one of a patient whose symptoms were aggravated because her psychiatrist put her under pressure to pray with her; one of a group of psychiatrists putting patients under pressure to engage in a political campaign; and one of a patient whose long-standing religious beliefs were denigrated by his psychiatrist. Soon after publication of these *Guidelines*, Marc Galanter (a member of the Committee on Religion and Psychiatry) published a report on the ways in which the clinical practice of 193 evangelical Christian psychiatrists was influenced by their religious beliefs (Galanter et al., 1991).

The *Guidelines* produced by the Committee on Religion and Psychiatry focussed on two concerns: maintaining of respect by psychiatrists for patients' beliefs, and not imposing psychiatrists' beliefs upon patients. In addressing the first of these concerns, it is positively affirmed that the taking of a history of patients' religious and other beliefs is 'useful', with a view to the possibility that they might be properly attended to in treatment. However, the emphasis is on respecting patients' vulnerabilities and on 'empathic respect for [the] value and meaning to the patient' of their beliefs (Committee on Religion and Psychiatry, 1990, p.542). In addressing the second concern, it is emphasised that religious concepts and rituals should not be employed in place of accepted psychiatric diagnoses and treatments.

The Joint Reference Committee of the APA updated this guidance in 2006 by way of a *Resource Document on Religious/Spiritual Commitments and Psychiatric Practice* (Peteet et al., 2006). In addition to the previous guidance, this document provided a third focus of concern, that 'Psychiatrists should foster recovery by making treatment decisions with patients in ways that respect and take into meaningful consideration their cultural, religious/spiritual, and personal ideals.' This positive recommendation included subclauses concerning the importance of spirituality/religion in relation to identity, hope, meaning and morality; 12-step programmes; mindfulness; the importance of spiritual/religious communities; and the importance of addressing differences in worldview between patients and psychiatrists early in treatment.

These guidelines were groundbreaking for psychiatry, both within the USA and internationally, and it is striking that there was apparently no attempt to produce similar guidance in other countries for at least a decade. It was only in 2005 that work began which led eventually to the publication of guidelines in the UK, and then internationally (Cook, 2017). Even then, the UK recommendations, approved by the Council of the Royal College of Psychiatrists, were not published until 2011 (Cook, 2011b).[2] Subsequently, national policies have been published by the South African Society of Psychiatrists (Janse Van Rensburg, 2014), the Canadian Psychiatric Association (CPA) (Chaimowitz et al., 2014), the Deutsche Gesellschaft für Psychiatrie und Psychotherapie, Psychosomatik und Nervenheilkunde (DGPPN) (Utsch et al., 2017) and the Royal Australian and New Zealand College of Psychiatrists (2018). Most recently, the Brazilian Psychiatric Association has

---

[2] Updated in 2013: Royal College of Psychiatrists, 2013.

commissioned the development of evidence-based guidelines for clinical practice, Part 1 of which was published in 2023 (Mosqueiro et al., 2023), with Part 2 expected in 2026. International guidance was approved by the Executive Committee of the WPA in 2015 (Moreira-Almeida et al., 2016) and has subsequently been translated into Portuguese, Spanish, French, Dutch, Arabic, Hindi and Chinese.

There is substantial overlap in recommendations made within these guidelines. Leaving aside for a moment the guidelines developed by the Brazilian Psychiatric Association, which are currently only partly published, all seven documents mention respect and/or sensitivity towards patients. Six out of seven have something to say about assessment, and not proselytising. These seem to be the core concerns. Four out of seven have something to say about training of psychiatrists, joint working with chaplains/clergy and treatment planning. Three mention research. There are various cross-references, and the development of these documents would seem to share a certain amount of common ground in terms of academic thought and international exchange.

A slightly different approach has been taken by the Brazilian Psychiatric Association, which has focussed on a systematic review process, Part 1 of which drew upon 6,609 articles, only 41 of which met all inclusion criteria. Two recommendations emerged from this substantial piece of work, the first of which was that a spiritual history should be taken routinely and as 'an essential part of the psychiatric interview' (Mosqueiro et al., 2023, p.515). The second was concerned with differentiating between 'cultural, anomalous, R/S experiences' and psychopathology (p.515). It is expected that Part 2 of the process will address integration of spirituality into clinical practice.

The document which stands out as most different from the others is that approved by the CPA's board of directors (Chaimowitz et al., 2014). Following the introduction and discussion, the statement made within this position statement affirms freedoms of conscience, religion and thought, 'sufficient that they should be able to communicate with and access psychiatric care free of religious ideas or belief systems foreign to them' (Chaimowitz et al., 2014, p.3). Finally, it affirms:

> For these reasons, we believe that psychiatric care, while sensitive to the spiritual, religious and cultural needs of the patient, needs to be provided in a secular fashion, attending to the best and most appropriate needs of the individual. It is important that psychiatrists, when they treat patients, do not allow their own religious beliefs or lack thereof to restrict or negatively affect the care they deliver to the patients that they serve and support. (p.3)

Whilst there is passing reference, in the introduction, to the wider debates on spirituality/religion in psychiatry, and it is conceded that 'This may be an important discussion' (Chaimowitz et al., 2014, p.2), this does not seem to be reflected in the conclusions. The emphasis is on prevention of abuse and the document seems to assume uncritically that this cannot (or is less likely to) occur in a secular context. It is neglectful of potential clinical benefits, seems to close down the 'important discussion' about spirituality/religion, rather than facilitating it, and provides no evidence base to support its conclusions.

A further Resource Document from the Joint Reference Committee of the APA, published in 2021, provides a longer, broader and updated discussion of the issues from a perspective south of the Canadian border (Dike et al., 2021). The guidelines of earlier documents are referenced but not repeated, and the conclusion states that 'The ethical boundaries in this area, as in many areas, cannot be reduced to absolute rules, but are best addressed by a commitment to the basic principles of providing compassionate, respectful, medically-appropriate care and avoiding gratifying the psychiatrist's needs or personal beliefs at the expense of the patient' (Dike et al., 2021, p.9). It is not clear whether this is intended to be a deliberate move away from rules and guidelines. Both the resource papers of the APA include a proviso that 'The findings, opinions, and conclusions of this report do not necessarily represent the views of the officers, trustees or all members of the American Psychiatric Association. Views expressed are those of the authors.' However, the affirmation of compassion and respect, and the acknowledgement of the importance of the boundary between the personal ('needs or personal beliefs') and the professional ('medically-appropriate') values of the psychiatrist effectively distil everything into three patient-centred principles: compassion, respect and an injunction against proselytising.

One of the key problems with guidelines and position statements (apart from the difficulty in reaching consensus) is that it is very hard to evidence the impact that they actually have (if any) upon clinical practice (Cook, 2017). It will be interesting to see what future developments emerge and whether research is able to provide any support for or against such initiatives. Meanwhile, important questions remain about how spirituality/religion are addressed in patient-centred psychiatric practice.

Secularity

It is notable that much of the debate amongst psychiatrists about spirituality and religion has taken place in the Western world. Apart from the guidelines from South Africa, all of the national guidelines referenced earlier come from North America, Europe, and Australia and New Zealand.[3] Similarly, published examples of boundary violations (see earlier) tend to come from Western countries. The national and international context of debate has therefore often reflected the concerns of secularism. As Charles Taylor has observed, secularism may mean different things (Taylor, 2007). In relation to psychiatry, it is importantly concerned with the way in which religious belief becomes merely one option amongst many.

In secular societies, the religious worldviews that historically provided meaning and purpose in life are contested. According to Taylor, various 'closed world structures' (CWSs) make disbelief seem much more incontrovertible than it actually is. Conversely, belief in a transcendent order is made to seem much less of an option than it actually is (Cook, 2010). Closed world structures, that is, 'ways of restricting our grasp of things which are not recognised as such' (Taylor, 2007, p.551), produce a loss of meaning, and a loss of transcendent reference, in secular society. Consequently, members of secular societies are 'cross-pressured', torn between belief and unbelief. The secular age in which we live is thus, Taylor says, suffering from a 'malaise of immanence' (Cook, 2012b) in which there is a bias against transcendent reference.

Secular space is not 'neutral' or 'safe' insofar as transcendence is concerned (Cook et al., 2011). The religious person is as likely to find himself/herself cross-pressured in a secular healthcare system as they may, for example, in a religious healthcare system of another tradition than their own. Indeed, the secular context may be even more threatening, by virtue of the CWSs that make it difficult to talk about religion at all. Some of the appeal of special interest groups for psychiatrists, such as SPSIG, may be that they provide a safe space

---

[3] The WPA position statement does reflect wider international debate, with authors from South America, South Africa and India, as well as Europe. However, this also draws on text from the UK RCPsych position statement.

within which such conversations may be had without fear of censure. Also, CWSs of this kind may explain why members of some Muslim communities are wary of accessing secular mental health services (Jafari, 1993; Weatherhead and Daiches, 2010).

The reality is that religion has not declined and disappeared as predicted by secularisation theory, and secular societies are having to accommodate religion, or at least spirituality, in a variety of ways. Amongst those who are not religiously affiliated (the so-called nones), a substantial proportion still hold spiritual beliefs of some kind (Evans et al., 2025a, 2025b). This recognition of the continuing presence of religion (or at least spirituality) in public life has been described as the post-secular, and it has important implications for psychiatry (Damberg Nissen et al., 2018). Psychiatry is faced with the challenge of renegotiating its relationship with religion and finding new and better ways of addressing the religiosity of patients in a post-secular world.

The CPA board of directors' statement that psychiatric care, 'while sensitive to the spiritual, religious and cultural needs of the patient, needs to be provided in a secular fashion, attending to the best and most appropriate needs of the individual' (Chaimowitz et al., 2014, p.3) is thus a complete non sequitur. If it is to be sensitive to the spiritual, religious and cultural needs of patients, psychiatric care needs to be provided not in 'a secular fashion' but in a compassionate, respectful and faith-affirming context. To this end, a non-secular (or perhaps post-secular) pluralism will usually be needed, in which the diversity of beliefs and worldviews that patients identify with is both recognised and affirmed. Psychiatric services need to be provided and delivered in such a way as to show respect for the different ways in which transcendence may be affirmed in support of mental well-being. Mental health and faith community partnerships (Perez et al., 2025), as promoted by the APA, might play a part in this, as might the willingness of psychiatric services to work collaboratively with faith-based organisations (Schumann et al., 2011) and mental health chaplains and spiritual care departments (Fletcher, 2019).

The aim, then, must be to be to create a safe space within which a patient can engage with all that might promote recovery. Despite all of the guidelines, the published debates and the examples of boundary violations, much less has been written about the nature of this safe space than one might have expected.

Temenos

In ancient Greek culture, a *temenos* (Zeiger, 2022) was a piece of land set apart and dedicated to a god. It could be a temple, for example, or a garden with a fountain, or a precinct. Jung adopted the term to refer to an inner sacred space – a safe space – in which spiritual transformation might take place. It is also used to refer to the place in which therapy might take place – although it is more a metaphorical place than a literal, physical one. It is safe because it has clear boundaries, and because of trust in the therapist, as much as being a safe physical location in which the therapist and the analysand might meet without interruption or interference.

What might the temenos for spirituality/religion in psychiatry look like? The temenos has many of the same qualities that Jeremy Holmes refers to as transitional space (see Chapter 3). However, I think that transitional space is just one way of conceiving of the temenos. In palliative care, the term has been used to refer to 'listening carefully to the patient, discerning what is of greatest importance, and fashioning a care plan that helps individuals and their loved ones achieve their ultimate goals' (Cook and Picchi, 2013, p.214).

Something similar would seem to be appropriate for psychiatry, and the language of 'greatest importance' and 'ultimate goals' has the benefit of not alienating those who find the language of spirituality/religion unhelpful. However, the concern here is with the way in which secularity can make it difficult to talk explicitly about spirituality/religion, and so these terms will be retained in the following discussion.

All of the position statements and guidelines cited earlier mention, in one way or another, the importance of respect for patients' spiritual/religious beliefs (and in some cases also those of colleagues). Words like trust, sensitivity, empathy and understanding are also used to expand upon, and qualify, the use of the word respect. The meaning of the word 'respect' appears to have changed over time and often now implies an emphasis on respect for autonomy rather than for humanity in general (Lysaught, 2004), a usage which endangers respect for those who (e.g., owing to intellectual disability or mental illness) have compromised autonomy. It is, however, a multifaceted concept which also includes such things as empathy, dignity, provision of information and attention to needs, and may have differently gendered emphases (Dickert and Kass, 2009). Speaking at a purely personal level, I would suggest that the core concept is not so much about autonomy as about respect for the common humanity that I share with my patient, and a humility about my own role in the therapeutic relationship.

One thing that almost everyone seems to agree on is that proselytising in the course of clinical practice is unethical. The temenos is not a place for proselytising; it is the very antithesis of this. Again, this is about respect and autonomy, but I think that the use of the word 'proselytising' is more problematic than it may appear to be. It has an implicitly negative nuance (Kerr, 1999). It might be seen as a kind of indoctrination, or perhaps as an unwanted conversation about religion, initiated for reasons that do not serve the best interests of the patient as understood from a patient-centred perspective. Similar concerns about proselytising arise with regard to other professional contexts where those cared for are vulnerable, for example as a result of age (Fagg, 2023). However, the term is often not defined, and it can sometimes be quite a subjective judgement as to what constitutes proselytising as opposed to a non-coercive, well-intentioned sharing of experience or information. The key concern in clinical psychiatry is that the power imbalance between doctor and patient, and the vulnerability of the patient, can easily render what might otherwise appear to be an innocent conversation completely inappropriate and abusive. The onus is therefore always on the psychiatrist to ensure that conversations about patients' religious beliefs (or lack of them) are not misinterpreted. Proselytising does not respect the autonomy of the patient and betrays a lack of humility on the part of the one doing the proselytising.

In contrast to the unwanted conversation that seeks to indoctrinate, the temenos for spirituality/religion in psychiatry fosters a safe place within which a patient may talk about the things that matter most to them – including belief, or non-belief, doubts, images of God, fears of evil, struggles in prayer and hopes for life after death. The content of such a conversation may be structured around a number of different published models of screening and assessment, or else may follow a more informal approach, but, however managed, it has to be non-intrusive and patient-centred.

In the RCPsych position statement (Royal College of Psychiatrists, 2013), it is pointed out that, in the course of clinical practice, a variety of attitudes to spirituality/religion may be encountered amongst patients (and colleagues), including

- identification with a particular social or historical tradition (or traditions)
- adoption of a personally defined, or personal but undefined, spirituality
- disinterest
- antagonism. (p.7)

The psychiatrist is unlikely to know in advance of meeting a new patient (or colleague) which of these attitudes to spirituality/religion they might have. Any opening question therefore needs to be non-directive and equally acceptable whether the attitude of the person concerned turns out to be one of antagonism or deeply held religious belief. The RCPsych information leaflet on spirituality and mental health suggests such initial questions as (amongst others) 'What is really important in your life?' or 'Would you say you are spiritual or religious in any way?', but each clinician may have their own preferences for how to open up the subject in a curious and patient-affirming way.

The temenos must be, therefore, a safe place. This is a basic requirement, but it is really only the starting point. The temenos should ideally facilitate (or at least not be a hindrance to) growth and transformation in every domain – biopsychosocial and spiritual. Where spiritual struggles are especially a focus of treatment, these may be dealt with in psychotherapy (Pargament and Exline, 2022). Spiritual concerns will also be addressed in many cases specifically in working with a mental health chaplain, spiritual director or faith leader. A variety of other spiritually integrated treatment options are also available, as discussed in Chapter 7.

Boundary-Building

The temenos becomes a safe space, at least in part, because it has clear boundaries, but these boundaries may be different for one patient and another, and (as we saw earlier) may be viewed very differently by one psychiatrist and another. Guidelines and position statements can go only so far and much remains very situational and specific to a particular patient, with particular concerns, in a therapeutic relationship with a particular psychiatrist. Given the complexity, controversy and sensitivity of the topic, what may be said about how psychiatrists may work together to create safely bounded temenoi for their patients?

This question may be answered at a variety of different levels, and I do not presume to have all of the answers. However, it seems to me that the starting point is to be able to continue a respectful, critical and constructive debate within the profession. This debate can – and should – take place in peer-reviewed journals, in conferences and in continuing professional development. It should be supported by empirical research. It needs to engage with sceptical voices, as well as with those who are like-minded, and it needs to include within its boundaries those who are agnostic, atheist and SBNR, as well as those who come from the world's major faith traditions. It needs to engage with the voices of patients and carers, as well as chaplains and faith leaders.

Within the context of this broader debate, there will also be a need for more special interest groups – temenoi for psychiatrists – within which there can be safe conversations amongst psychiatrists who want to talk about spirituality, including their own spiritualities and their patients' spiritualities, in relation to clinical practice. If we cannot talk safely with one another about these things, it is unlikely that we will be able to talk safely with our patients about them. If I can talk respectfully with my colleague, who shares my perspective that spirituality is important but whose spirituality is very different from mine, then I am better equipped to care well for the patient whose spirituality is different from mine. In the course of these conversations with my colleagues, I also learn a lot about my own spirituality, as I am questioned about it and it is reflected back to me. In this way, I experience opportunities for spiritual growth, which, in turn, broadens my perspective and makes me less likely to inadvertently impose my unexamined spiritual preconceptions upon my patients.

At a third level of answering my question, there will be the boundaries that protect each individual clinical consultation, some of which are very general (as in guidelines and position statements) but some of which will be very particular to a given patient or situation. Ideally, these might be negotiated explicitly with a patient – as in asking the question 'Would you like to discuss this further?' – but in other cases they may remain implicit. Good psychiatrists are used to creating safe spaces within which, when necessary, they can discuss sensitive topics that are open to potential misunderstanding, such as sexuality, relationships, trauma and abuse. The skills that enable these other sensitive conversations to be conducted within safe boundaries are transferrable to conversations about spirituality/religion.

There are, however, at least two more levels at which to consider this question of how to build good boundaries. Crucially, there is that aspect of the temenos which is bounded not externally, by the clinical consultation, but internally, within the mind of the patient. This is the inner sacred space within which Jung understood the potential for spiritual transformation. What goes on in this space – between a soul and God, one might say, but perhaps using other language – operates within the boundaries of the psyche. It is a place within which unconscious material may come to the fore and present challenging existential and spiritual questions about interpretation and meaning which need to be subjected to careful discernment. The most important thing here will be for the psychiatrist not to get in the way of what is going on spiritually, but that is not to say that these things will not be discussed, especially in dynamic psychotherapy, where a patient may want to talk about them. These are the things that many patients will also want to discuss with a priest, chaplain, spiritual director or other spiritual/religious confidant. Some patients have written eloquently about the spiritual transformations that have taken place in the context of their mental illness (see, for example, Murphy, 2010; Barber, 2016; Hastings, 2020).

Correspondingly, the practice of psychiatry raises boundary questions for the psychiatrist – as in my story of my own experiences, related in Chapter 2. Here, and in contrast to what goes on in the clinical interaction between patient and psychiatrist, the boundaries of professional and personal values are necessarily broken down and subject to critical examination. My spirituality affects how I practise psychiatry, and the study and practice of psychiatry affects my spirituality, in a two-way interaction which can be either positive or negative, for my patients and for me. The better able I am to examine these dynamics within the safe boundaries of supervision, a peer group or spiritual direction, the better able I will be to provide safe boundaries for my patients.

Psychiatrists and Spirituality

Is it ever permissible for a psychiatrist to pray with his or her patient? I have heard it said that this should be a clear boundary, and that guidelines should include injunctions against it. It was one of the hot topics in the published debate following the publication of Harold Koenig's controversial editorial in *Psychiatric Bulletin* in 2008 (Koenig, 2008b). At the end of this chapter, however, I'd like to reverse the question. Is it ever permissible for a psychiatrist *not* to pray with his or her patient?

Clearly, the answer to this question is yes – of course it is – especially when that prayer is out loud and in circumstances where a patient does not want this, or where a psychiatrist has no faith and does not believe in prayer. To expect prayer in such circumstances would be a violation of the temenos, that sacred space which a psychiatrist has a duty to respect and protect in the course of patient-centred practice. In fact, a violation of this kind would not really be prayer at all. It would be spiritual abuse. True prayer (as explored in Chapter 7) is something very different from this – concerned with giving careful attention to relationships between the human person and a transcendent order – however understood.

What about a situation in which a patient requests prayer from their psychiatrist, and the patient and psychiatrist share the same faith tradition? This would be more complicated, especially if the psychiatrist was providing psychotherapy to the patient, and especially if what is meant is prayer spoken out loud in the clinic. However, a respect for the sanctity of the temenos, and for the autonomy of the patient, might also make this difficult to refuse. Indeed, there is a broader issue here about what prayer might mean (as explored in Chapter 7) that might make a refusal difficult to justify ethically, theologically, psychologically and spiritually. Such a refusal might be a violation of the patient's temenos, a lack of humility on the part of the psychiatrist and a harmful intrusion of secularity into clinical practice.

Then again, if (as Simone Weil proposed – see Chapter 7) 'Absolutely unmixed attention is prayer' (Weil, 1952, p.106), anything less than this on the part of a psychiatrist will always be less than any patient has a right to expect from their psychiatrist. Keeping spirituality in mind in this way is simply good psychiatry.

I suppose that I am being rather mischievous in making this proposal, and I do it only to try to help clarify the issues at hand. The CWSs that operate in secular society make it seem 'obvious' that prayer with a patient might be a breach of professional boundaries, in ways that would seem completely unobvious to people who do not live within the CWSs of secularity. It is because of these CWSs that secularity is not experienced as a safe space for those who identify as spiritual/religious. For the religious person (patient or psychiatrist) for whom prayer is part of the very fabric of life, injunctions not to pray, especially when this is usually only silently, are intrusive and unethical. Secularity, in its more aggressive forms, seems to demand that everyone adopt a pragmatic atheism when seeing their doctor. However, we are now in a post-secular world. What is really needed is a safe place within which psychiatrists and patients can be authentically themselves, including their spiritual selves, in a respectful and patient-centred way.

Conclusions

Psychiatry with Spirituality in Mind

As we come to the end of this book, what conclusions might we draw about spirituality and psychiatry? What does psychiatry look like in the light of spirituality?

Spirituality and psychiatry are entangled. They are mixed up and intertwined in all kinds of ways, implicitly or explicitly, in theory and in practice: in healthy mental processes and in psychopathology; in the minds of psychiatrists and patients; in the very nature of the concepts of spirituality, religion and psychiatry; in the complex relationships between science and theology, and psychiatry and religion; in clinical practice; and – most importantly of all – in the lives of patients. The fact that there has been so much effort invested in trying to disentangle them, almost always to the detriment of patients, actually only serves to highlight the extent to which they are in practice inseparable.

The concept of entanglement, as articulated by Fitzgerald and Callard (2016), has two parts to it. Firstly, there is the reference to a 'set of things, commonly held to be separate from one another (indeed, that define themselves precisely with reference to their separability)', for which Fitzgerald and Callard give as examples 'science and justice, humans and non-humans, settlers and natives' (p.39). Then, secondly, there is the realisation that this set of things 'not only might have something in common, but also, in fact, may be quite *inseparable* from one another' (Fitzgerald and Callard, 2016, p.39). In application to psychiatry, I am proposing that spirituality and psychiatry (a) are commonly held to be separate and define themselves precisely with reference to their separability, and (b) not only have something in common but are in fact quite inseparable. Having spent the last eight chapters exploring some particular aspects of this tangle, I'd now like to map out the more general nature of what I am proposing.

Two Proposals

I imagine that my first proposal, that spirituality and psychiatry are commonly held to be separate, is unlikely to be contentious. I think that most people see them as completely separate, and possibly even in opposition to each other. Psychiatry as a domain of research and academic endeavour is concerned with science and objectivity. As a product of Enlightenment rationality, it puts behind it (what might be perceived to be) the superstitions and myths belonging to an enchanted universe that humankind has now allegedly outgrown. As clinical practice, psychiatry is primarily concerned with mental illness and not with matters of spirituality or faith. There are disciplinary boundaries to be observed and these clearly exclude things like theology, spirituality and religion from the purview of psychiatry. Psychiatry, anxious even within the world of medicine to demonstrate its legitimacy, increasingly tends to emphasise neuroscience and biology as the basis for its professional credibility.

Those who identify as spiritual or religious (especially if they do not have a psychiatric diagnosis themselves) may also have good reasons to see psychiatry as something completely separate from the worlds of faith, theology and spirituality. The latter are concerned with a transcendent order, not amenable to scientific verification or disproof, and they are concerned with a different understanding of what it is to be human than that provided by the neurosciences or the social sciences. They may also be somewhat sensitive to a perception that psychiatry has historically been rather hostile to religion, diagnosing spiritual or religious beliefs as pathology rather than recognising them as a basis for human flourishing. With a heartfelt vision of what it is to live a good life, spirituality decries the view that only science can tell us what is real. It is primarily concerned with human flourishing, not with mental illness.

I think that there are therefore good grounds for proposing that spirituality and psychiatry comprise a 'set of things' commonly held to be separate. As will probably be obvious by now to readers who have followed my line of argument through this book, this set of things also includes some other things, things which overlap conceptually with either spirituality or psychiatry, or both. These other things include theology, religion and secularity. Even though spirituality and religion are conceptually separate, for many people they overlap considerably in practice, whereas for others they are seen as being in opposition to each other. Theology and religious studies have their own contradistinctions, reflecting different stances on what it is to be objective, and the extent to which distancing oneself from the object of study might be helpful. Secularity, as we have seen in earlier chapters, has a complex relationship with both spirituality and religion, keeping the latter separate from itself to a greater extent than the former, but also providing the social and cultural context within which psychiatry is usually practised (at least in the Western world). Whilst acknowledging all of this, I'm bracketing these things out for a moment, so as to focus on the alleged separateness of spirituality and psychiatry. Keeping them in mind, I realise that the separateness that I am portraying here is somewhat of an oversimplification. Nonetheless, I contend that it does lay behind the debates about the extent to which spirituality can be, or properly should not be, brought into the practice of psychiatry. Spirituality and psychiatry are commonly perceived to be separate things; they should be kept apart, it is said, and they need boundaries to keep them apart.

My second proposal is that spirituality and psychiatry actually have a lot in common and, in fact, are inseparable. They are both concerned with the human condition, albeit these concerns have different objectives in mind. Spirituality is concerned with a broad view of human relationships, incorporating both transcendent and immanent dimensions, and with finding meaning and purpose. Psychiatry is concerned in clinical practice with the relief of mental suffering and, in support of this, with a biopsychosocial framework of understanding how human beings function. However, both are concerned with all the things that make us uniquely human, our thoughts and feelings, how we behave and what motivates us, our deepest desires, our relationships and our perception of our place in the world around us. Both are concerned with the relief of human distress and with what religion sometimes calls the 'cure of souls'. Psychiatry has traditionally been less concerned with finding existential or spiritual meaning in life but, as we have seen earlier in the book, it has the potential to contribute significantly to this quest (or else to hinder it).

Whilst spirituality and psychiatry have a lot in common, my main contention here is not so much to map the boundaries of their respective concerns as to argue that they are in practice inseparable, at least if psychiatry is to live up to its aspiration of offering a person-centred holistic model of care. The case study with which I opened this book, in Chapter 1, demonstrates that neglect of this inseparability risks failure to properly understand exactly what it is that is causing our patients distress and prejudices our ability to offer a complete and maximally effective treatment plan. As I outlined in Chapter 2, the thinking of psychiatrists has long entangled their views about spirituality, theology and religion with their views about psychiatry, and it is better to acknowledge this than to try to disentangle them (which is probably impossible anyway). Most importantly, in Chapter 3, my argument was that spirituality is inextricably entangled with the concerns of psychiatry in the minds of patients. To try to disentangle at this level is fundamentally in contradiction to the aspirations of the person-centred holistic model of psychiatry. It risks imposing a secular and atheistic worldview which is hostile and antipathetic to the spiritual concerns that many patients find central to their self-identity and well-being.

More Tangles

In broader terms, psychiatry is caught up in debates about the relationship between science and theology. Whereas a lot of consideration has been given to this interdisciplinary engagement in relation to, for example, cosmology, quantum physics and evolution (see, for example, Polkinghorne, 1998; McGrath, 2009; Northcott and Berry, 2009), relatively little attention has been given to the relationship insofar as it affects psychiatry. In Chapter 4, I considered some of the ways in which theology – what I am calling clinical theology – might better inform a person-centred, holistic approach to psychiatry. Clinical theology of the kind that I am envisaging does not impose formal or normative theologies (or atheologies) but, rather, seeks to understand the ways in which the ordinary theologies of patients are entangled with their insight into their spiritual condition and the psychopathology of their illnesses.

Spirituality and psychiatry are perhaps most obviously entangled in relation to psychopathology, and, in Chapter 5, I explored the ways in which this entanglement might present in relation to the phenomenon of auditory verbal hallucinations. In a longer work, such entanglements might have been explored also in relation to other aspects of mental state, such as affect, thought disorder and hallucinations in other modalities. When psychiatry has acknowledged a kind of entanglement of spirituality/religion with psychopathology, it has tended to respond by trying to disentangle, to undertake a differential diagnosis that will distinguish between 'valid' spiritual experience and illness (see, for example, Moreira-Almeida, 2009). What is needed is not disentanglement (which is impossible anyway) but an affirmation that psychopathology is inseparable from spirituality in many cases, and that the spiritual aspects of psychopathology can be meaningful and are an important part of illness experience for patients. They are also an important basis from which to develop the spiritual dimensions of a treatment plan.

Some of the entanglements that present a particular challenge to patients and others are those that might be grouped under the heading of spiritual struggles, or the related concept, negative religious coping. In Chapter 6, I explored one particular kind of spiritual struggles, demonic struggles, in relation to a patient who presented complaining that he was possessed by evil spirits. For this patient, it was not just the inseparability of spirituality/religion and phenomenology that was a challenge but also, and more importantly, the way in which spirituality was entangled with his efforts to explain what was happening to him and to cope with the significant psycho-spiritual stresses that he was experiencing at the time.

Sometimes, spirituality is a significant part of the clinical problem but – at the same time – this provides opportunities to reimagine treatment planning in such a way as to encourage positive spiritual coping and turn these concerns to therapeutic advantage.

Spirituality is also inseparable from (at least some of) the positive coping mechanisms that might promote recovery. One of the topics that has provoked most controversy in relation to spirituality and psychiatry (as discussed in Chapter 8) has been that of praying with patients. At the same time, one of the spiritual interventions that has gained widest acceptance has been mindfulness. Prayer, mindfulness and silence (the focus of Chapter 7) are all practices in which spirituality is inseparable from the psychological task of giving careful attention. Each has its own evidence base, but each also highlights the paradox that it is not a utilitarian focus on outcomes that matters most (especially where outcomes are conceived in reductionistic and purely scientific terms), so much as the way in which we give careful, compassionate attention to the human condition, both our own and that of our patients. In planning treatment in psychiatry, it is fundamental that we consider carefully the choice of things that we give attention to, and the quality of attention that we give to them.

The Quest for Meaning

Helping patients to find meaning in the context of their mental illnesses has not traditionally been seen as part of psychiatry, but meaning-making is a core part of what it is to be human and is beneficial to mental health (Egnew, 2009; Steger, 2022). It doesn't matter too much whether we call this a spiritual quest or not, but for most people worldwide it does take on spiritual or religious forms. As we have seen earlier in the book, meaning-making has historically taken a wide variety of forms in the thinking of both psychiatrists and their patients. It has the potential to provide a positive coping resource for patients in the process of recovery. Why, then, has it not featured more prominently in psychiatric training and practice?

I suspect that the answer to this is, to a large extent, buried in the history of psychiatry as it was born and established in the context of Enlightenment rationalism and the scientific perspectives emphasised and affirmed by Henry Maudsley and others. It has been reinforced by the closed world structures (CWSs) of secularism (as discussed in Chapters 1 and 8) which relegate religion to a private sphere and exclude it from the public square. If we try to stand back from these CWSs which, as Taylor (2007) emphasises, seem so normal to us now that they are virtually invisible, it does nonetheless seem very odd. Why should I not be able to discuss my spiritual/religious concerns with a psychiatrist, given that I can discuss just about anything else with him/her and that such concerns are so completely inseparable from the biopsychosocial framework to which mental health professionals give such careful attention? Is it the case that psychiatrists are really supposed to imagine that life is meaningless, or that they cannot help – in a patient-centred way – with the spiritual quest to find meaning amidst illness? To put the question slightly differently, taking up Jenny's words (from the case study in Chapter 1), 'Is nothing sacred?' If the answer that psychiatry gives is 'No – nothing is sacred', then it has completely lost touch with the things that matter most to the majority of its patients. It is also completely out of touch with a post-secular world.

Clearly chaplaincy and spiritual care teams have a lot to contribute in this patient-led quest for meaning (Fletcher, 2019), as do local faith communities, and the task at hand is a collaborative one, not something that will be undertaken by psychiatrists in isolation from others. However, the psychiatrist who does not convey to his or her patients an understanding of the importance of this task risks undermining the therapeutic alliance, conveying a lack of empathy and presenting a less than human face to those who come to them in search of help.

One of my key conclusions in this book is that psychiatry needs to look for ways in which the search for meaning, not to mention spirituality more broadly, can be brought centre stage in clinical practice and training. This is not a paradigm shift. It is simply taking seriously what psychiatry already aspires to, but often fails to deliver, in the context of a truly person-centred holistic model of practice. It requires much more attention to the humanities, including theology and spiritual/religious studies, in the course of psychiatric training and continuing professional development.

Undoing the Damage

Contemporary psychiatry has inherited an unfortunate history of antagonism towards spirituality/religion which has inhibited engagement of those who identify as spiritual/religious with psychiatric services and has made them wary of discussing their concerns with their psychiatrist when they do. It has prevented psychiatrists, when developing a treatment plan with and for their patients, from recognising important resources available to promote spiritual coping and recovery. Hopefully, the Freudian days of seeing religion as part of the problem are over, but there is still damage to be undone. Psychiatry must find ways of conveying the message to patients that it can offer safe spaces within which to discuss their spiritual/religious concerns and that it sees these as positive resources for recovery which are to be welcomed and affirmed. How might this be done?

Firstly, and most importantly, within clinical consultations, psychiatrists need to communicate to patients, when and where appropriate, that spirituality is affirmed as being importantly and positively interconnected with mental well-being. If a spiritual assessment is conducted with sensitivity and care, then this will usually be implicit. However, it will also need to be made explicit, by showing interest in spiritual/religious matters raised by patients, by encouraging them to say more about these concerns, by offering referral to the chaplaincy or spiritual care team and by flagging spiritual practices, where helpful to do so, as components of a holistic treatment plan. Psychiatrists also need to be aware of various forms of pathological spirituality which may be harmful to mental health, to have the skills to deal with these sensitively and to refer appropriately to colleagues who specialise in helping patients to recover from the harm that they cause.

Secondly, there is a need to build good working partnerships with faith communities. The model of mental health and faith community partnerships adopted by the American Psychiatric Association (Idler et al., 2019; Perez et al., 2025) is one which has much to offer in the UK and in other countries. Closer local working relationships between faith communities and NHS mental health trusts are needed, as a basis for establishing trust and mutual understanding. At the same time, national and international initiatives, such as those promoted by the Spirituality and Psychiatry Special Interest Group (SPSIG) or the World Psychiatric Association (WPA) Section on Religion and Spirituality, have the potential to raise the profile and understanding of these issues amongst psychiatrists and, indirectly, the wider population.

Faith communities have a responsibility to provide better training of clergy and faith leaders in relation to mental health and in reducing the stigma associated with psychiatry and mental illness. It is part of the professional role of psychiatrists to assist in this educational endeavour. Mental health also needs to be seen as a concern in relation to interfaith dialogue, where we all have much to learn from each other in promoting mutual understanding of the barriers that prevent people of many different faiths from finding the help that they need when suffering from mental illness.

Boundaries

As I outlined in Chapter 8, I do believe that boundaries are important in psychiatry, not least in relation to spirituality and religion. However, it is important to recognise that such boundaries are necessarily created and imposed. They do not represent any kind of naturally occurring discontinuity between the things that they separate. Spirituality and psychiatry are – as I proposed earlier – inseparable. This makes boundaries all the more important. They are needed not to keep out of practice things that are central to good practice but to create safe spaces – temenoi – within which psychological and spiritual transformations can occur. These spiritual processes potentially take place within all of the domains with which psychiatry is inherently concerned – the biological, the psychological and the social – and are inseparable from this biopsychosocial matrix.

The boundaries that I have in mind exclude secularity from clinical interactions because its CWSs can be just as damaging, if not more so, than any of the abuses of religion or spirituality that have taken place in clinical practice. The temenos that I am envisaging as central to good psychiatric practice is not secular space, at least not for most patients; it is post-secular. It is a patient-centred spiritual space within which healing and transformation can take place. It has boundaries, but they are not boundaries between the secular and the religious, and they are not boundaries of specialist expertise. To the extent that they are boundaries between the personal and professional lives of the psychiatrist, they are semi-permeable because it is important that the humanity of the psychiatrist should not be excluded from this sacred space.

As discussed in Chapter 8, such boundaries are not easily condensed into succinct guidelines for good practice. Whilst I believe that we do need guidelines, and there are some basic things that can be said to help prevent repetition of some of the more egregious abuses that have occurred in the past, and to affirm basic tenets of good practice, there is much that is more situational in nature and open to legitimate professional debate. Much more research is needed on the ways in which psychiatrists manage these boundaries in practice, and on how we might manage them better.

Clinical Theology

The kind of clinical theology that I am proposing in this book is very different from that which Frank Lake had in mind in his book of that name. Firstly, and most importantly, it is not a confessional theology but an inclusive one, more a kind of respectful listening than a profession of knowledge. Secondly, it is not primarily a formal theology but, rather, a thoughtful attentiveness to the ordinary theology of patients as it informs their insight into their condition and as may be relevant to an holistic understanding of the genesis, development and treatment of mental disorders. Thirdly, it draws quite widely on other disciplines, notably the study of religion and the study of spirituality, but also the humanities more widely. I hope that the importance of this kind of clinical theology has already become clear in the case studies of Jenny (Chapter 1), Hannah (Chapter 3), Amir (Chapter 5) and Alejo (Chapter 6), not to mention my own story (Chapter 2). There are many further avenues of clinical theology of this kind which we might have explored in this book, and which deserve further attention in clinical practice. It is not possible to explore them all here, but I will mention just two as worthy of further consideration.

Reincarnation

Belief in reincarnation is widespread around the globe (Evans et al., 2025b), including in European countries (Haraldsson, 2013), as well as in the United States (Walker, 2000; Alper et al., 2023). It is traditionally associated with Asian religious traditions such as Hinduism and Buddhism but is also common amongst those who self-identify as spiritual but not religious (SBNR). Reincarnation is important for psychiatry because of the ways in which it influences clinician and patient understandings of the causes of psychopathology.

Reincarnation, also known as rebirth, metempsychosis or transmigration, concerns a belief that there is a continuity of some kind (a self, or soul or consciousness) from one life to the next (Bowker, 1999). Usually, this continuity is understood as being between successive human lives, but in Hinduism there is also a belief in the possibility of rebirth as an animal. Belief in reincarnation is commonly linked with, but distinct from, belief in karma, a law of consequences whereby rebirth in the next life is understood as linked to moral behaviour in the present life.

In past-life regression therapy (PLR) (Cook, 2022a, p.382), therapeutically induced regression (e.g., under hypnosis) is used to recover alleged memories of past lives. There are numerous case reports according to which PLR is highly effective. For example, Alan Sanderson describes a patient who, under hypnosis, when asked to go back to the onset of his depression and anxiety, 'went back' to a time when he was a Roman solider dying in combat (Sanderson, 2023). There seems to be general agreement amongst advocates that, some of the time, false memories are generated. For believers in reincarnation, the question arises of how true and false memories might be distinguished. However, alternative explanations abound, including notably false memory syndrome, cryptomnesia, social construction of memories, confabulation, fantasy and (according to Jungian analysts) recovery of memories from a collective unconscious. Thus, PLR is controversial, and there is a substantial body of opinion that identifies PLR as discredited and unethical (Norcross et al., 2006; Thomason, 2010).

Why do I mention this controversial topic here? Firstly, it challenges me, as a Christian psychiatrist who does not believe in reincarnation, to reflect on how I have managed significant theological differences that may have existed between me and my patients. I like to think that I have always been respectful of my patients' beliefs and that I have encouraged open discussion, where relevant to my professional role, however implausible my patient's beliefs might have seemed to me. However, I can't remember a patient ever telling me that they believe in reincarnation, and I am left wondering why. Statistically, I must have had patients who believed in reincarnation. Did they not feel able to discuss this with me? Was it not seen as relevant by my patients, so they didn't mention it? Have I simply forgotten what they told me? I am reminded that listening well is an active process and that sometimes we need to go out of our way to ensure that our patients feel free to discuss with us – if they want to – things that they might feel are 'out of bounds' to psychiatry.

Secondly, there is evidence that beliefs in reincarnation may be associated with higher rates of common mental disorders and post-traumatic stress disorder (PTSD) (Carvalho et al., 2025), a history of survival of violent trauma (Davidson et al., 2005) and anxiety (Gadit, 2009). In a study of children who report past-life memories, gender non-conformity was more common amongst those whose birth sex was different in the reported past life (Pehlivanova et al., 2018). In certain cultural contexts, reincarnation is sometimes thought to offer an explanation of the cause of mental disorders (Daie, 1992; Wynaden et al., 2005; Igberase and Okogbenin, 2017). There is an empirical body of evidence, some of it contributed by psychiatrists, in support of reincarnation (Moreira-Almeida et al., 2022). It is an important part of evidence-based psychiatry to be aware of this literature and to take it into account in clinical practice, even if we might have a variety of different interpretations of it. (I am not personally persuaded by the evidence in support of reincarnation, but I respect others who take a different view from mine.)

Thirdly, it is always important to understand our patients' stories in spiritual and religious context. Given that belief in reincarnation is so prevalent, a better understanding of such beliefs seems to me to be an important part of patient-centred psychiatry. It highlights a challenge in relation to how we manage the religiosity gap between psychiatrist/therapist and patient (Peres, 2012). In an age of trauma-informed practice (Isobel et al., 2021), it is important to be informed about ordinary theologies of trauma.

I recognise that this is a controversial example, and I would not personally be happy to work with PLR therapy. However, it is illustrative of the complexity of issues that might arise, theologically and scientifically, when addressing the entanglements of spirituality and psychiatry in clinical practice.

Atheologies

As will have been clear through earlier chapters of this book, the so-called nones, those who answer negatively in response to questionnaires about religious identity and affiliation, are a very heterogeneous group. Quite apart from those who identify as SBNR, including some who might identify with an atheistic spirituality, there are those who would see themselves as 'agnostic' in some broad sense (not necessarily in the strict philosophical sense of the word) and those who would identify as atheist by conviction. A belief that there is no God or gods is a particular theological worldview and may be significant in terms of its implications for finding meaning and purpose in life.

I remember with some sadness a patient who described himself as an atheist, married to a practising Catholic. I had treated him for a diagnosis of depressive disorder. He had recovered from his illness, having made a good response to treatment, but I had continued to see him in the outpatient clinic as he wanted to continue to discuss his struggles around finding meaning and purpose in life as an atheist. He was jealous of his wife's faith, in terms of the certainties that it seemed to offer her, but he could not share her beliefs. One day, I was not there when he attended the clinic, and he was discharged by a colleague. In one sense, this was a completely correct clinical decision. He had made a good clinical recovery. In another sense, it left some important psychological and spiritual loose ends which were highly relevant to future prognosis and relapse prevention. A few weeks later, he was found dead in a remote spot in the countryside where he had gone to take his own life. I can't be sure that this wouldn't still have happened if he had seen me again in the clinic, or if he hadn't been discharged from the clinic, but it still left me with a regret that I hadn't been there for him at that last outpatient appointment. For me, it was a harsh reminder not only that spirituality matters but that meaning and purpose matter for all of us, atheists included.

For many, atheism and agnosticism are much more settled systems of belief and there is evidence that firm convictions, of this kind may even benefit mental health, to a degree comparable with that of religious belief, as compared with other forms of what we might call more 'unsettled' unbelief (Galen and Kloet, 2010; Moore and Leach, 2016; Baker et al., 2018; Gontijo et al., 2022). The outpatient clinic is categorically not a place for proselytising. However, it is a place for exploring the ways in which spirituality and ordinary theology influence mental well-being.

By 'ordinary theology', it is important to recognise that – in terms of the clinical theology that I am proposing – there might be a very wide range of theologies and atheologies, and of intellectual rigour and knowledge. Theologians and clergy are not immune to mental ill health, just as atheists are not necessarily predisposed to it. Clinical theology is concerned with emotional regulation, spiritual coping and spiritual struggles in relation to an almost limitless spectrum of beliefs and unbeliefs.

The Gaps in This Book

This book has not been completely comprehensive, and I have been deliberately and necessarily selective in the examples that I have used to paint a picture of how I think a person-centred holistic model of psychiatry can be attentive to spirituality, religion and clinical theology. Before I close, it seems appropriate to flag up some of the omissions.

Some of the gaps arise simply because this is a book by only one psychiatrist, writing from a particular cultural perspective, at a particular point in time. Some of the gaps in this book are attended to in other, multi-author books such as *Spirituality and Psychiatry* (Cook and Powell, 2022). However, I think we also need more books by those who write from different personal perspectives of spirituality, religion or history than mine. In this book I deliberately avoided Christian theology as much as possible, in order that I could write for a wider audience, but we do need books that explore Christian, Muslim, Hindu and other theologies, critically and in depth. Although I have highlighted the importance of what I have called clinical theology, it ended up being only a small part of this book and I think there is much more to be said about the ways in which the ordinary theologies of patients (and clinicians) impact upon their understandings of health and illness.

The shape of this book was sketched out in such a way as to paint a picture of spirituality in psychiatry as a whole, but I think we also need much more attention to the phenomenology and theology of particular diagnostic categories such as depression, anxiety, trauma-related diagnoses and the various kinds of psychosis. Experiences such as the 'dark night of the soul' in Christianity (Cook, 2024a) and Kundalini awakening in Eastern faith traditions (Fonteijn, 2020) have largely been explored in the past from theological and religious perspectives, but they overlap considerably with the concerns of psychiatry and we need more interdisciplinary, empirical and theological engagement with the kinds of psycho-spiritual struggle that they represent.

Historically, psychiatry has operated from the basis of a scientific anthropology which has been attentive to mind and body. It has more recently, creatively and constructively, been enriched by engagement with cultural anthropology, and there is scope for it to be even further enriched by engagement with theological anthropologies, and with the broader field of the critical medical humanities. A holistic model of psychiatry needs to be much more attentive to the full range of academic and lay perspectives on what it is to be human.

Spiritually Attentive Psychiatry

I have been arguing that psychiatrists need to keep spirituality in mind in the course of their clinical practice. Spirituality seeks to give attention to core human concerns, including relationships and meaning and purpose in life. For many it is fundamentally about attending to a transcendent order, however conceived, although there are in fact forms of spirituality which focus more on the immanent than on the transcendent (Cook, 2013c). Mindfulness is an example of an immanently focussed spiritual practice. In either case, it gives attention to 'something more', variously defined in a multitude of person-centred ways.

Religion also has its core concerns, overlapping heavily with those of spirituality for most people. The 'building blocks' of religion, as described by Anne Taves (2011), focus attention on certain 'special things', notably anomalous things (with or without agency) and ideal things. Whereas religion, like much of spirituality, has a focus on the transcendent, it is also very concerned with the immanent order.

Psychiatry, in apparent contrast to all of this, focusses its attention on mental illness but, as Nancy Andreasen (1997) and others have pointed out, mental illness is different from other kinds of illness because of the ways in which minds create humanity and shape our sense of identity. Psychiatry cares for people whose illnesses affect the very core of their existence, and thus their spirituality and their religious faith. It has the potential to assist in the crucial process of finding meaning amidst illness and adversity in ways which can be highly complementary to those provided by spirituality and religion.

If psychiatry is spiritually inattentive, if psychiatrists do not keep spirituality in mind, then people will seek help elsewhere. If psychiatry has not built good partnerships with communities and organisations that are able to positively affirm the connections between spirituality and mental health, then patients will seek help from spiritual sources that may be inattentive to mental health concerns, or even psychologically harmful. There are therapists, healers, exorcists and others who, adopting a model of antagonism between the worlds of spirituality and psychiatry, will readily offer inappropriate, harmful and ill-advised interventions to those who seek their help in this way. Spiritual practitioners are not regulated in the way that medical professionals are, and those who suffer from mental disorders are vulnerable to exploitation by them.

I am concerned here not only with what we give attention to but also with the quality of attention that we give. There is a quality of attentiveness which might be described as 'spiritual', regardless of whether it is focussed on doing a jigsaw puzzle (I was working on a jigsaw whilst writing some of the chapters of this book) or seeing a patient in the clinic. It is in the nature of human attentiveness that we are easily distracted, by both internal stimuli (thoughts, mental images, memories) and external stimuli (perceptions). However, we can choose to be attentive to a particular thing – and to keep bringing our attention back when it wanders (e.g., as in mindfulness) – and we can be captivated by something such that our attention does not wander (e.g., as in some mystical experiences or 'flow' experiences). Prayer, mindfulness and silence each bring their own opportunities to develop a quality of attentiveness, to a valued focus of attention, in such a way that we might call it 'spiritual'.

What kind of attentiveness is it that we offer, then, when – as psychiatrists – we see a patient in the clinic or on the ward? We have all struggled, when on call late at night, or when preoccupied with worries of our own, to give the kind of attention that we would ideally like to offer to every patient. Making the choice, if necessary repeatedly and frequently, to turn our attention back to our patient and to give them our best attention is both a professional duty and a spiritual practice. Spirituality is deeply entangled with psychiatric practice, even if we choose to call it by another name. Spiritually attentive psychiatrists enter into patients' experiences of what it is to be human by way of being fully attentive to their own humanity.

Chiaroscuro

I began, in the Introduction to this book, with a metaphor of light and shadow. This arose partly in response to the title of Tom Burns's book, in which he refers to psychiatry as 'our necessary shadow' (Burns, 2014). This in turn evokes a reminder of the importance of the concept of the shadow as understood in Jungian analytical psychology. For Jung, the process of individuation involved an assimilating into consciousness of those aspects of ourselves which we find unacceptable, uncomfortable or frightening. In this process, paradoxically, we discover that the dark and shadowy side of Self contains much that is illuminating and healing. Psychiatrists and their patients, through vocation or illness, find themselves immersed in this world of the interplay between metaphorical light and darkness, themes which also have great significance in theology and spirituality.

Elsewhere, under the title of 'Chiaroscuro' (Cook, 2025a), I wrote about how my own experiences around the time of my wife's death impacted upon my practice as a psychiatrist and my thinking about faith in relation to psychiatry. In the world of art, the term chiaroscuro refers to the interplay of light and dark in a painting or photograph. This interplay has long fascinated me, both as an amateur photographer and as someone who enjoys art. In my early training as a psychiatrist, participating in an art therapy group led by my colleagues in occupational therapy, I discovered that visual images often enabled my patients to talk about things that were otherwise too difficult to articulate, to explore the metaphorical shadows, psychological and spiritual, that were otherwise too painful to think about. Psychiatry, then, is not so much about our necessary shadow (although, in Jungian terms, that is one of its key concerns) as it is about the light that it throws in its therapeutic endeavour to address the suffering associated with mental illness. A kind of psycho-spiritual chiaroscuro emerges in the pictures of life that are painted by psychiatrists and their patients as they are faced with the tensions between what they most fear and what they most deeply desire.

References

Abdulkerim, N. & Li, C. (2022) How Applicable Are Mindfulness-Based Interventions to Muslim Clients in the US? *Professional Psychology: Research and Practice*, **53**, 253–265.

Abu-Raiya, H., Pargament, K. I., Exline, J. J. & Agbaria, Q. (2015a) Prevalence, Predictors, and Implications of Religious/Spiritual Struggles among Muslims. *Journal for the Scientific Study of Religion*, **54**, 631–648.

Abu-Raiya, H., Pargament, K. I., Weissberger, A. & Exline, J. (2015b) An Empirical Examination of Religious/Spiritual Struggle among Israeli Jews. *International Journal for the Psychology of Religion*, **26**, 61–79.

Achour, M., Muhamad, A., Syihab, A. H., Mohd Nor, M. R. & Mohd Yusoff, M. Y. Z. (2021) Prayer Moderating Job Stress among Muslim Nursing Staff at the University of Malaya Medical Centre (UMMC). *Journal of Religion and Health*, **60**, 202–220.

Adityanjee, M. D., Raju, G. S. P. & Khandelwal, S. K. (1989) Current Status of Multiple Personality Disorder in India. *American Journal of Psychiatry*, **146**, 1607–1610.

Adshead, G. & Horne, E. (2021) *The Devil You Know: Stories of Human Cruelty and Compassion*. London: Faber.

Aguilar, M. I. (2017) *The Way of the Hermit: Interfaith Encounters in Silence and Prayer*. London: Jessica Kingsley.

Aizik-Reebs, A., Shoham, A. & Bernstein, A. (2021) First, Do No Harm: An Intensive Experience Sampling Study of Adverse Effects to Mindfulness Training. *Behaviour Research and Therapy*, **145**, 103941.

Al-Krenawi, A. & Graham, J. R. (1997) Spirit Possession and Exorcism in the Treatment of a Bedouin Psychiatric Patient. *Clinical Social Work Journal*, **25**, 211–222.

Al-Krenawi, A. & Graham, J. R. (2000) Islamic Theology and Prayer: Relevance for Social Work Practice. *International Social Work*, **43**, 289–304.

Aldbyani, A. (2024) Exploring Islamic Mindfulness: Cultural Practices and Their Impact on Public Health Outcomes. *Mindfulness*, **16**, 695–701.

Alderson-Day, B. (2023) *Presence: The Strange Science and True Stories of the Unseen Other*. Manchester: Manchester University Press.

Ali, A. Y. (2000) *The Holy Qur'an: Translation and Commentary*. Birmingham: IPCI (Islamic Presentation Centre International) Islamic Vision.

Ali, M. (2014) Perspectives on Drug Addiction in Islamic History and Theology. *Religions*, **5**, 912–928.

Ali, M. M. (2015) Praying Alongside Patients: Personal Reflections on Therapeutic Supplications. *Journal of Spirituality in Mental Health*, **17**, 187–189.

Allport, G. W. & Ross, J. M. (1967) Personal Religious Orientation and Prejudice. *Journal of Personality and Social Psychology*, **5**, 432–443.

Alper, B. A., Rotolo, M., Tevington, P., Nortey, J. & Kallo, A. (2023) *Spirituality among Americans*. Pew Research Center, 7 December. www.pewresearch.org/religion/2023/12/07/spirituality-among-americans/.

American Psychiatric Association (2013) *Diagnostic and Statistical Manual of Mental Disorders, Fifth Edition (DSM-5)*. Washington, DC: American Psychiatric Association.

American Psychiatric Association (n.d.) Mental Health and Faith Community Partnership. www.psychiatry.org/psychiatrists/diversity/mental-health-and-faith-community-partnership.

Anderson, J. W. & Nunnelley, P. A. (2016) Private Prayer Associations with Depression, Anxiety and Other Health Conditions: An

Analytical Review of Clinical Studies. *Postgraduate Medicine*, **128**, 635–641.

Anderson, N., Heywood-Everett, S., Siddiqi, N., Wright, J., Meredith, J. & McMillan, D. (2015) Faith-Adapted Psychological Therapies for Depression and Anxiety: Systematic Review and Meta-analysis. *Journal of Affective Disorders*, **176**, 183–196.

Andreasen, N. C. (1997) What Is Psychiatry? *American Journal of Psychiatry*, **154**, 591–593.

Antic, A. (2021) Transcultural Psychiatry: Cultural Difference, Universalism and Social Psychiatry in the Age of Decolonisation. *Culture, Medicine, and Psychiatry*, **45**, 359–384.

Argyle, M. (2002) State of the Art: Religion. *The Psychologist*, **15**, 22–26.

Ascoli, M., Palinski, A., Abdul-Hamid, W. K. & Dein, S. (2014) Cultural Consultation for Jinn and Spirit Possession in Muslim Psychiatric Patients: A Case Series. *World Cultural Psychiatry Research Review*, **June**, 65–69.

Aslan, R. (2011) *No God but God: The Origins, Evolution, and Future of Islam*. New York: Random House.

Astley, J. & Francis, L. J. (2013) *Exploring Ordinary Theology*. Farnham: Ashgate.

Baccetto, L. (2023) Spiritualizing Psychiatry: Transpersonal Psychology, DSM, and Brazilian Research about Spirituality. *Social Compass*, **70**, 481–497.

Back, A. L., Bauer-Wu, S. M., Rushton, C. H. & Halifax, J. (2009) Compassionate Silence in the Patient–Clinician Encounter: A Contemplative Approach. *Journal of Palliative Medicine*, **12**, 1113–1117.

Bade, M. K. & Cook, S. W. (2008) Functions of Christian Prayer in the Coping Process. *Journal for the Scientific Study of Religion*, **47**, 123–133.

Baer, R., Crane, C., Montero-Marin, J., Phillips, A., Taylor, L., Tickell, A., Kuyken, W. & Team, M. (2021) Frequency of Self-Reported Unpleasant Events and Harm in a Mindfulness-Based Program in Two General Population Samples. *Mindfulness (N Y)*, **12**, 763–774.

Baesler, E. J. & Ladd, K. (2009) Exploring Prayer Contexts and Health Outcomes: From the Chair to the Pew. *Journal of Communication and Religion*, **32**, 347–374.

Baetz, M., Griffin, R., Bowen, R. & Marcoux, G. (2004) Spirituality and Psychiatry in Canada: Psychiatric Practice Compared with Patient Expectations. *Canadian Journal of Psychiatry*, **49**, 265–271.

Bagasra, A. (2023) Religious Interpretations of Mental Illness and Help-Seeking Experiences among Muslim Americans: Implications for Clinical Practice. *Spirituality in Clinical Practice*, **10**, 20–31.

Bailey, E. (2010) Implicit Religion. *Religion*, **40**, 271–278.

Baker, J. O., Stroope, S. & Walker, M. H. (2018) Secularity, Religiosity, and Health: Physical and Mental Health Differences between Atheists, Agnostics, and Nonaffiliated Theists Compared to Religiously Affiliated Individuals. *Social Science Research*, **75**, 44–57.

Banks, R. (1973) Religion as Projection: A Re-appraisal of Freud's Theory. *Religious Studies*, **9**, 401–426.

Bänziger, S., Janssen, J. & Scheepers, P. (2008a) Praying in a Secularized Society: An Empirical Study of Praying Practices and Varieties. *International Journal for the Psychology of Religion*, **18**, 256–265.

Bänziger, S., Uden, M. V. & Janssen, J. (2008b) Praying and Coping: The Relation between Varieties of Praying and Religious Coping Styles. *Mental Health, Religion and Culture*, **11**, 101–118.

Barber, J. (2016) My Story: A Spiritual Narrative. In Cook, C. C. H., Powell, A. & Sims, A. (Eds.), *Spirituality and Narrative in Psychiatric Practice: Stories of Mind and Soul*. London: Royal College of Psychiatrists, 121–131.

Barber, J. (2022) The Patient Perspective. In Cook, C. C. H. & Powell, A. (Eds.), *Spirituality and Psychiatry*. Cambridge: Cambridge University Press, 293–311.

Barber, J. M., Parsons, H., Wilson, C. A. & Cook, C. C. H. (2017) Measuring Mental Health in the Clinical Setting: What Is

Important to Service Users? The Mini-Service User Recovery Evaluation Scale (Mini-SeRvE). *Journal of Mental Health*, **26**, 530–537.

Barbour, I. G. (1998) *Religion and Science*. London: SCM.

Barlow, D. H., Abel, G. G. & Blanchard, E. B. (1977) Gender Identity Change in a Transsexual: An Exorcism. *Archives of Sexual Behavior*, **6**, 387–395.

Barrett, J. L. & Keil, F. C. (1996) Conceptualizing a Nonnatural Entity: Anthropomorphism in God Concepts. *Cognitive Psychology*, **31**, 219–247.

Bassett, L., Bingley, A. F. & Brearley, S. G. (2018) Silence as an Element of Care: A Meta-ethnographic Review of Professional Caregivers' Experience in Clinical and Pastoral Settings. *Palliative Medicine*, **32**, 185–194.

Basu, S., Gupta, S. C. & Akthar, S. (2002) Trance and Possession Like Symptoms in a Case of CNS Lesion: A Case Report. *Indian Journal of Psychiatry*, **44**, 65–67.

Batson, C. D. (1976) Religion as Prosocial: Agent or Double Agent? *Journal for the Scientific Study of Religion*, **15**, 29–45.

Bayer, R. S. & Shunaigat, W. M. (2002) Sociodemographic and Clinical Characteristics of Possessive Disorder in Jordan. *Neurosciences*, **7**, 46–49.

Beck, R. & Taylor, S. (2008) The Emotional Burden of Monotheism: Satan, Theodicy, and Relationship with God. *Journal of Psychology and Theology*, **36**, 151–160.

Bergunder, M. (2014) What Is Religion? The Unexplained Subject Matter of Religious Studies. *Method and Theory in the Study of Religion*, **26**, 246–286.

Berry, R. J. (2007) *Creation and Evolution Not Creation or Evolution*. Cambridge: Faraday Institute for Science and Religion.

Beyers, J. (2022) Feuerbach, Religion and Post-Theism. *HTS Teologiese Studies / Theological Studies*, **78**, a7781.

Bhugra, D. & Ventriglio, A. (2015) Social Sciences and Medical Humanities: The New Focus of Psychiatry. *BJPsych (British Journal of Psychiatry) International*, **12**, 79–80.

Bhui, K., King, M., Dein, S. & O'Connor, W. (2009) Ethnicity and Religious Coping with Mental Distress. *Journal of Mental Health*, **17**, 141–151.

Bingaman, K. A. (2003) *Freud and Faith: Living in the Tension*. New York: State University of New York Press.

Black, S. W., Pössel, P., Jeppsen, B. D., Tariq, A. & Rosmarin, D. H. (2015) Poloma and Pendleton's (1989) Prayer Types Scale in Christian, Jewish, and Muslim Praying Adults: One Scale or a Family of Scales? *Psychology of Religion and Spirituality*, **7**, 205–216.

Bockrath, M. F., Pargament, K. I., Wong, S., Harriott, V. A., Pomerleau, J. M., Homolka, S. J., Chaudhary, Z. B. & Exline, J. J. (2022) Religious and Spiritual Struggles and Their Links to Psychological Adjustment: A Meta-Analysis of Longitudinal Studies. *Psychology of Religion and Spirituality*, **14**, 283–299.

Boelens, P. A., Reeves, R. R., Replogle, W. H. & Koenig, H. G. (2009) A Randomized Trial of the Effect of Prayer on Depression and Anxiety. *International Journal of Psychiatry in Medicine*, **39**, 377–392.

Boelens, P. A., Reeves, R. R., Replogle, W. H. & Koenig, H. G. (2012) The Effect of Prayer on Depression and Anxiety: Maintenance of Positive Influence One Year after Prayer Intervention. *International Journal of Psychiatry in Medicine*, **43**, 85–98.

Bolwig, T. G. (2006) Psychiatry and the Humanities. *Acta Psychiatrica Scandinavica*, **114**, 381–383.

Bonchek, A. & Greenberg, D. (2009) Compulsive Prayer and Its Management. *Journal of Clinical Psychology*, **65**, 396–405.

Bonelli, R. M. & Koenig, H. G. (2013) Mental Disorders, Religion and Spirituality 1990 to 2010: A Systematic Evidence-Based Review. *Journal of Religion and Health*, **52**, 657–673.

Bose, R. (1997) Psychiatry and the Popular Conception of Possession among the Bangledeshis in London. *International Journal of Social Psychiatry*, **43**, 1–15.

Bourguignon, E. (Ed.) (1973) *Religion, Altered States of Consciousness, and Social Change*. Columbus: Ohio State University Press.

Bourguignon, E. (1976) *Possession*. San Francisco, CA: Chandler and Sharp.

Bourguignon, E. (1978) Spirit Possession and Altered States of Consciousness: The Evolution of an Inquiry. In Spindler, G. D. (Ed.), *The Making of Psychological Anthropology*. Berkeley: University of California Press, 479–515.

Bowker, J. (1999) *The Oxford Dictionary of World Religions*. Oxford: Oxford University Press.

Bowman, E. S. (1993) Clinical and Spiritual Effects of Exorcism in Fifteen Patients with Multiple Personality Disorder. *Dissociation*, **VI**, 222–238.

Bracken, P., Thomas, P., Timimi, S., Asen, E., Behr, G., Beuster, C., Bhunnoo, S., Browne, I., Chhina, N., Double, D., Downer, S., Evans, C., Fernando, S., Garland, M. R., Hopkins, W., Huws, R., Johnson, B., Martindale, B., Middleton, H., Moldavsky, D., Moncrieff, J., Mullins, S., Nelki, J., Pizzo, M., Rodger, J., Smyth, M., Summerfield, D., Wallace, J. & Yeomans, D. (2012) Psychiatry beyond the Current Paradigm. *British Journal of Psychiatry*, **201**, 430–4.

Bradshaw, M., Ellison, C. G. & Flannelly, K. J. (2008) Prayer, God Imagery, and Symptoms of Psychopathology. *Journal for the Scientific Study of Religion*, **47**, 644–659.

Bradshaw, M., Ellison, C. G. & Marcum, J. P. (2010) Attachment to God, Images of God, and Psychological Distress in a Nationwide Sample of Presbyterians. *International Journal for the Psychology of Religion*, **20**, 130–147.

Bravesmith, A. (2012) Silence Lends Integrity to Speech: Transcending the Opposites of Speech and Silence in the Analytic Dialogue. *British Journal of Psychotherapy*, **28**, 21–34.

Breslin, M. J. & Lewis, C. A. (2008) Theoretical Models of the Nature of Prayer and Health: A Review. *Mental Health, Religion and Culture*, **11**, 9–21.

Britton, W. B., Lindahl, J. R., Cooper, D. J., Canby, N. K. & Palitsky, R. (2021) Defining and Measuring Meditation-Related Adverse Effects in Mindfulness-Based Programs. *Clinical Psychological Science*, **9**, 1185–1204.

Brown, D. W. (2009) *A New Introduction to Islam*. Oxford: Wiley-Blackwell.

Bull, D. L., Ellason, J. W. & Ross, C. A. (1998) Exorcism Revisited: Positive Outcomes with Dissociative Identity Disorder. *Journal of Psychology and Theology*, **26**, 188–196.

Bullivant, S. (2017) *The 'No Religion' Population of Britain*. London: St Mary's University.

Bullough, V. L. (1985) Spirit Rapping Unmasked: An 1851 Investigation and Its Aftermath. *The Skeptical Inquirer*, **10**, 60–67.

Burns, T. (2014) *Our Necessary Shadow*. London: Penguin.

Burton, L. (2015) Prayers on a Prayer Tree: Ordinary Theology from a Tourist Village. *Rural Theology*, **8**, 62–77.

Bussema, E. F. & Bussema, K. E. (2007) Gilead Revisited: Faith and Recovery. *Psychiatric Rehabilitation Journal*, **30**, 301–5.

Butler, B. & Butler, T. (1996) *Just Spirituality in a World of Faith*. London: Mowbray.

Cain, C. D. (2019) The Effects of Prayer as a Coping Strategy for Nurses. *Journal of Perianesthesia Nursing*, **34**, 1187–1195.

Callard, F. & Margulies, D. S. (2014) What We Talk about When We Talk about the Default Mode Network. *Frontiers in Human Neuroscience*, **8**, 619.

Cameron, H., Bhatti, D., Duce, C., Sweeney, J. & Watkins, C. (2010) *Talking about God in Practice: Theological Action, Research and Practical Theology*. London: SCM.

Campbell, A. V. (2019) Cult Books Revisited: Frank Lake's Clinical Theology. *Theology*, **122**, 164–171.

Canby, N. K., Cosby, E. A., Palitsky, R., Kaplan, D. M., Lee, J., Mahdavi, G., Lopez, A. A., Goldman, R. E., Eichel, K., Lindahl, J. R. & Britton, W. B. (2025) Childhood Trauma and Subclinical PTSD Symptoms Predict Adverse Effects and Worse Outcomes across Two Mindfulness-Based Programs for Active Depression. *PLoS One*, **20**, e0318499.

Captari, L. E., Hook, J. N., Hoyt, W., Davis, D. E., McElroy-Heltzel, S. E. & Worthington, E. L., Jr (2018) Integrating Clients' Religion and Spirituality within

Psychotherapy: A Comprehensive Meta-analysis. *Journal of Clinical Psychology*, **74**, 1938–1951.

Cardeña, E. (2023) The Other in the Self: Possession, Trance, and Related Phenomena. In Dorahy, M. J., Gold, S. N. & O'Neil, J. A. (Eds.), *Dissociation and the Dissociative Disorders: Past, Present, Future*. New York: Routledge, 421–432.

Carrette, J. & King, R. (2005) *Selling Spirituality: The Silent Takeover of Religion*. London: Routledge.

Carson, V. B. & Koenig, H. G. (2004) *Spiritual Caregiving: Healthcare as Ministry*. Philadelphia, PA: Templeton.

Carvalho, S. M. d., Tucker, J., Moreira-Almeida, A. (2025) Who Does Report Past-Life Memories? Claimers' Profile, Religiosity/Spirituality and Impact on Happiness and Mental Health. *International Journal for the Psychology of Religion*, **35**(4), 285–300.

Casher, M. I. (2013) 'There's No Such Thing as a Patient': Reflections on the Significance of the Work of D. W. Winnicott for Modern Inpatient Psychiatric Treatment. *Harvard Review of Psychiatry*, **21**, 181–7.

Cave, B. (2023) *What We Fear Most: A Psychiatrist's Journey to the Heart of Madness*. London: Seven Dials.

Chaimowitz, G., Urness, D., Mathew, B., Dornik, J. & Freeland, A. (2014) Freedom of and from Religion. *Canadian Journal of Psychiatry*, **59**, 1–3.

Chandrashekar, C. R., Chaonabasavaona, S. M. & Reddy, M. V. (1980) Hysterical Possession Syndrome: A Retrospective Study. *Indian Journal of Psychological Medicine*, **3**, 35–40.

Chapin, D. (2000) The Fox Sisters and the Performance of Mystery. *New York History*, **81**, 157–188.

Chatterjee, P. (2012) On Being a Patient. *International Journal of User-Driven Healthcare*, **2**, 57–59.

Cheyne, J. A. (2012) Sensed Presences. In Blom, J. D. & Sommer, I. E. C. (Eds.), *Hallucinations: Research and Practice*. New York: Springer, 219–234.

Chur-Hansen, A. & Parker, D. (2005) Is Psychiatry an Art or a Science? The Views of Psychiatrists and Trainees. *Australasian Psychiatry*, **13**, 415–418.

Clare, A. (1980) *Psychiatry in Dissent: Controversial Issues in Thought and Practice*. London: Routledge.

Clark, D. A., Abramowitz, J., Alcolado, G. M., Alonso, P., Belloch, A., Bouvard, M., Coles, M. E., Doron, G., Fernández-Álvarez, H., Garcia-Soriano, G., Ghisi, M., Gomez, B., Inozu, M., Moulding, R., Radomsky, A. S., Shams, G., Sica, C., Simos, G. & Wong, W. (2014) Part 3. A Question of Perspective: The Association between Intrusive Thoughts and Obsessionality in 11 Countries. *Journal of Obsessive-Compulsive and Related Disorders*, **3**, 292–299.

Clarke, I., Mottram, K. & Taylor, S. (2016) Narratives of Transformation in Psychosis. In Cook, C. C. H., Powell, A. & Sims, A. (Eds.), *Spirituality and Narrative in Psychiatric Practice*. London: Royal College of Psychiatrists, 108–120.

Clements, A. D. & Ermakova, A. V. (2012) Surrender to God and Stress: A Possible Link between Religiosity and Health. *Psychology of Religion and Spirituality*, **4**, 93–107.

Cocksworth, A. (2023) When Prayer Goes Wrong: A Negative Theology of Prayer. *Scottish Journal of Theology*, **76**, 10–23.

Colman, W. (2006) The Self. In Papadopoulos, R. (Ed.), *The Handbook of Jungian Psychology*. London: Routledge, 153–174.

Committee on Religion and Psychiatry (1990) Guidelines Regarding Possible Conflict between Psychiatrists' Religious Commitments and Psychiatric Practice. *American Journal of Psychiatry*, **147**, 542.

Cook, C. C. H. (1985) Leukaemia in the Family. *British Medical Journal*, **291**, 1810–1811.

Cook, C. C. H. (2004) Addiction and Spirituality. *Addiction*, **99**, 539–551.

Cook, C. C. H. (2006) *Alcohol, Addiction and Christian Ethics*. Cambridge: Cambridge University Press.

Cook, C. C. H. (2010) Spirituality, Secularity and Religion in Psychiatric Practice. *The Psychiatrist*, **34**, 193–195.

Cook, C. C. H. (2011a) The Faith of the Psychiatrist. *Mental Health, Religion and Culture*, **14**, 9–17.

Cook, C. C. H. (2011b) *Recommendations for Psychiatrists on Spirituality and Religion*. London: Royal College of Psychiatrists.

Cook, C. C. H. (2012a) Healing, Psychotherapy, and the *Philokalia*. In Bingaman, B. & Nassif, B. (Eds.), *The Philokalia: A Classic Text of Orthodox Spirituality*. Oxford: Oxford University Press, 230–239.

Cook, C. C. H. (2012b) Self-Belief: Holistic Psychiatry in a Secular Age. Commentary on . . . Holistic Psychiatry without the Whole Self. *The Psychiatrist*, **36**, 101–103.

Cook, C. C. H. (2013a) Controversies on the Place of Spirituality and Religion in Psychiatric Practice. In Cook, C. C. H. (Ed.), *Spirituality, Theology and Mental Health*. London: SCM, 1–19.

Cook, C. C. H. (Ed.) (2013b) *Spirituality, Theology and Mental Health*. London: SCM.

Cook, C. C. H. (2013c) Transcendence, Immanence and Mental Health. In Cook, C. C. H. (Ed.), *Spirituality, Theology and Mental Health*. London: SCM, 141–159.

Cook, C. C. H. (2015) Religious Psychopathology: The Prevalence of Religious Content of Delusions and Hallucinations in Mental Disorder. *International Journal of Social Psychiatry*, **61**, 404–425.

Cook, C. C. H. (2017) Spirituality and Religion in Psychiatry: The Impact of Policy. *Mental Health, Religion and Culture*, **20**, 589–594.

Cook, C. C. H. (2018) *Hearing Voices, Demonic and Divine: Scientific and Theological Perspectives*. London: Routledge.

Cook, C. (2020a) Psychiatric Training – Looking Back. *The Registrar*, **October**, 14–16.

Cook, C. C. H. (2020b) Spirituality, Religion and Mental Health: Exploring the Boundaries. *Mental Health, Religion and Culture*, **23**, 363–374.

Cook, C. C. H. (2020c) What Did Jesus Have to Say about Mental Health? In Cook, C. C. H. & Hamley, I. (Eds.), *The Bible and Mental Health: Towards a Biblical Theology of Mental Health*. London: SCM, 128–140.

Cook, C. C. H. (2022a) Glossary. In Cook, C. C. H. & Powell, A. (Eds.), *Spirituality and Psychiatry*, 2nd ed. Cambridge: Cambridge University Press, 375–400.

Cook, C. C. H. (2022b) Leah's Voices: Reflections on Auditory Verbal Hallucinations as Spiritual and Religious Experience. In Woods, A., Alderson-Day, B. & Fernyhough, C. (Eds.), *Voices in Psychosis: Interdisciplinary Perspectives*. Oxford: Oxford University Press, 176–183.

Cook, C. C. H. (2022c) Preface to the Second Edition. In Cook, C. C. H. & Powell, A. (Eds.), *Spirituality and Psychiatry*. Cambridge: Cambridge University Press, xi–xii.

Cook, C. C. H. (2022d) Religion and Religious Experience. In Cook, C. C. H. & Powell, A. (Eds.), *Spirituality and Psychiatry*, 2nd ed. Cambridge: Cambridge University Press, 312–331.

Cook, C. C. H. (2022e) Spirituality and Religion in Psychiatry. In Cook, C. C. H. & Powell, A. (Eds.), *Spirituality and Psychiatry*. Cambridge: Cambridge University Press, 1–22.

Cook, C. C. H. (2023a) *Hearing Spiritual Voices: Medieval Mysticism, Meaning and Psychiatry*. London: T&T Clark.

Cook, C. C. H. (2023b) Theology and Psychiatry. In Wolfe, B. N. (Ed.), *St Andrews Encyclopaedia of Theology*. St Andrews: University of St Andrews.

Cook, C. C. H. (2024a) The Dark Night in Psychiatry. In Howells, E. & Tyler, P. (Eds.), *John of the Cross: Carmel, Desire and Transformation*. London: Routledge, 249–262.

Cook, C. C. H. (2024b) Deliverance in Practice: Mental Health, Theology and Professional Boundaries. In Strawbridge, J., Adams, N. & Hamley, I. (Eds.), *Deliver Us from Evil: Church, Theology and Deliverance Ministry*. London: SCM, 51–69.

Cook, C. C. H. (2025a) Chiaroscuro. In Roberts, G. (Ed.), *Personally Speaking*. Independently published, 59–65.

Cook, C. C. H. (2025b) Demon Possession, Theology, and Mental Health. *Journal of Disability and Religion*, **29**, 171–189.

Cook, E. & Picchi, C. (2013) The Temenos of Palliative Care. *Psychological Perspectives*, **56**, 212–220.

Cook, C. C. H. & Powell, A. (Eds.) (2022) *Spirituality and Psychiatry*. Cambridge: Cambridge University Press.

Cook, C. C. H. & White, N. H. (2018) Resilience and the Role of Spirituality. In Bhugra, D., Bhui, K., Yeung, S., Wong, S. & Gilman, S. E. (Eds.), *Oxford Textbook of Public Mental Health*. Oxford: Oxford University Press, 513–520.

Cook, C. C. H., Powell, A., Sims, A. & Eagger, S. (2011) Spirituality and Secularity: Professional Boundaries in Psychiatry. *Mental Health, Religion and Culture*, **14**, 35–42.

Cook, C. C. H., Breckon, J., Jay, C., Renwick, L. & Walker, P. (2012) Pathway to Accommodate Patients' Spiritual Needs. *Nursing Management*, **19**, 33–37.

Cook, C. C. H., Powell, A. & Sims, A. (Eds.) (2016) *Spirituality and Narrative in Psychiatric Practice: Stories of Mind and Soul*. London: Royal College of Psychiatrists.

Cook, C. C. H., Powell, A., Alderson-Day, B. & Woods, A. (2022) Hearing Spiritually Significant Voices: A Phenomenological Survey and Taxonomy. *BMJ (British Medical Journal) Medical Humanities*, **48**, 273–284.

Cook, C. C. H., Hamley, I. & Swinton, J. (2023) *Struggling with God: Mental Health and Christian Spirituality*. London: SPCK.

Cook, C. C. H., Francis, L. J. & Village, A. (2025) Psychological Temperament and Augustinian Prayer and Spirituality: A Replication Study. *Journal of Spiritual Formation and Soul Care*.

Coons, P. M. (1993) The Differential Diagnosis of Possession States. *Dissociation*, **VI**, 213–221.

Cottam, S., Paul, S. N., Doughty, O. J., Carpenter, L., Al-Mousawi, A., Karvounis, S. & Done, D. J. (2011) Does Religious Belief Enable Positive Interpretation of Auditory Hallucinations? A Comparison of Religious Voice Hearers with and without Psychosis. *Cognitive Neuropsychiatry*, **16**, 403–421.

Cowden, R. G., Pargament, K. I., Chen, Z. J., Davis, E. B., Lemke, A. W., Glowiak, K. J., Rueger, S. Y. & Worthington, E. L. Jr (2022) Religious/Spiritual Struggles and Psychological Distress: A Test of Three Models in a Longitudinal Study of Adults with Chronic Health Conditions. *Journal of Clinical Psychology*, **78**, 544–558.

Crichton, P., Carel, H. & Kidd, I. J. (2017) Epistemic Injustice in Psychiatry. *BJPsych Bulletin*, **41**, 65–70.

Crowley, N. & Jenkinson, G. (2022) Pathological Spirituality. In Cook, C. C. H. & Powell, A. (Eds.), *Spirituality and Psychiatry*. Cambridge: Cambridge University Press, 332–354.

Culliford, L. (2002) Spiritual Care and Psychiatric Treatment: An Introduction. *Advances in Psychiatric Treatment*, **8**, 249–261.

Culliford, L. (2011a) Beware! Paradigm Shift under Way. *Mental Health, Religion and Culture*, **14**, 43–51.

Culliford, L. (2011b) *The Psychology of Spirituality*. London: Jessica Kingsley.

Cullinan, R. J., Woods, A., Barber, J. M. P. & Cook, C. C. H. (2024) Spiritually Significant Hallucinations: A Patient-Centred Approach to Tackle Epistemic Injustice. *BJPsych Bulletin*, **48**, 133–138.

Currier, J. M., Foster, J. D., Abernethy, A. D., Witvliet, C. V. O., Root Luna, L. M., Putman, K. M., Schnitker, S. A., Vanharn, K. & Carter, J. (2017) God Imagery and Affective Outcomes in a Spiritually Integrative Inpatient Program. *Psychiatry Research*, **254**, 317–322.

Daie, N. (1992) The Belief in the Transmigration of Souls: Psychotherapy of a Druze Patient with Severe Anxiety Reaction. *British Journal of Medical Psychology*, **65**, 119–130.

Dalrymple, W. (2009) *Nine Lives: In Search of the Sacred in Modern India*. London: Bloomsbury.

Damberg Nissen, R., Gildberg, F. & Hvidt, N. (2018) Psychiatry, a Secular Discipline in a Postsecular World? A Review. *Religions*, **9**, article 32.

Darwin, C. ([1859] 1998) *The Origin of Species*. Ware: Wordsworth Editions.

Datta, V. (2016) Humanities More Important Than Ever in the Era of Scientific Psychiatry. *American Journal of Psychiatry Residents' Journal*, **11**, 2.

David, A. S. (2004) The Cognitive Neuropsychiatry of Auditory Verbal Hallucinations: An Overview. *Cognitive Neuropsychiatry*, **9**, 107–123.

Davidson, J. R., Connor, K. M. & Lee, L. C. (2005) Beliefs in Karma and Reincarnation among Survivors of Violent Trauma – A Community Survey. *Social Psychiatry and Psychiatric Epidemiology*, **40**, 120–125.

Davis, E. B., Moriarty, G. L. & Mauch, J. C. (2013) God Images and God Concepts: Definitions, Development, and Dynamics. *Psychology of Religion and Spirituality*, **5**, 51–60.

De Brito Sena, M. A., Damiano, R. F., Lucchetti, G. & Peres, M. F. P. (2021) Defining Spirituality in Healthcare: A Systematic Review and Conceptual Framework. *Frontiers in Psychology*, **12**, 756080.

De Haan, S. (2021) Bio-psycho-social Interaction: An Enactive Perspective. *International Review of Psychiatry*, **33**, 471–477.

Dein, S. & Cook, C. C. H. (2015) God Put a Thought into My Mind: The Charismatic Christian Experience of Receiving Communications from God. *Mental Health, Religion and Culture*, **18**, 97–113.

Dein, S. & Littlewood, R. (2008) The Psychology of Prayer and the Development of the Prayer Experience Questionnaire. *Mental Health, Religion and Culture*, **11**, 39–52.

Delaruelle, J. (2003) Attention as Prayer: Simone Weil. *Literature and Aesthetics*, **13**, 19–27.

De Leede-Smith, S. & Barkus, E. (2013) A Comprehensive Review of Auditory Verbal Hallucinations: Lifetime Prevalence, Correlates and Mechanisms in Healthy and Clinical Individuals. *Frontiers in Human Neuroscience*, **7**, 367.

De Menezes, A. & Moreira-Almeida, A. (2009) Differential Diagnosis between Spiritual Experiences and Mental Disorders of Religious Content. *Revista de Psiquiatria Clínica*, **36**, 69–76.

Dennett, D. C. (1991) *Consciousness Explained*. London: Penguin.

De Villaine, H. (2020) Explaining Religion by Human Faculties: The Naturalism of Henry Maudsley. *International Journal of Philosophy and Theology*, **81**, 369–385.

Dickert, N. W. & Kass, N. E. (2009) Understanding Respect: Learning from Patients. *Journal of Medical Ethics*, **35**, 419–23.

Dike, C., Briz, L., Fadus, M., Martinez, R., May, C., Milone, R., Nesbit-Bartsch, A., Powell, T., Witmer, A. & Weintraub Brendel, R. (2021) *Resource Document on Ethics at the Interface of Religion, Spirituality, and Psychiatric Practice*. Washington, DC: American Psychiatric Association.

Donahue, M. J. (1985) Intrinsic and Extrinsic Religiousness: Review and Meta-analysis. *Journal of Personality and Social Psychology*, **48**, 400–419.

Donelli, D., Lazzeroni, D., Rizzato, M. & Antonelli, M. (2023) Silence and Its Effects on the Autonomic Nervous System: A Systematic Review. *Progress in Brain Research*, **280**, 103–144.

Dossett, W. (2015) Reflections on the Language of Salvation in Twelve-Step Recovery. In Bacon, H., Dossett, W. & Knowles, S. (Eds.), *Alternative Salvations*. London: Bloomsbury, 21–30.

During, E. H., Elahi, F. M., Taieb, O., Moro, M.-R. & Baubet, T. (2011) A Critical Review of Dissociative Trance and Possession Disorders: Etiological, Diagnostic, Therapeutic, and Nosological Issues. *Canadian Journal of Psychiatry*, **56**, 235–242.

Edwards, D. (1999) *The God of Evolution*. New York: Paulist Press.

Egnew, T. R. (2009) Suffering, Meaning, and Healing: Challenges of Contemporary Medicine. *Annals of Family Medicine*, **7**, 170–5.

Eguchi, S. (1991) Between Folk Concepts of Illness and Psychiatric Diagnosis: Kitsune-Tsuki (Fox Possession) in a Mountain Village of Western Japan. *Culture, Medicine and Psychiatry*, **15**, 421–451.

Engel, G. L. (1977) The Need for a New Medical Model: A Challenge for Biomedicine. *Science*, **196**, 129–136.

Enoch, D. (2006) *I Want a Christian Psychiatrist*. Oxford: Monarch.

Enoch, D., Puri, B. K. & Ball, H. (2021) *Uncommon Psychiatric Syndromes*. Oxford: Routledge.

Enoch, M. D. & Trethowan, W. H. (1979) *Uncommon Psychiatric Syndromes*. Bristol: Wright.

Epstein, M. (2013) *The Trauma of Everyday Life*. Carlsbad, CA: Hay House.

Epstein, M. (2022) *The Zen of Therapy: Uncovering a Hidden Kindness in Life*. New York: Penguin.

Escolà-Gascón, Á., Ovalle, M. & Matthews, L. (2023) Interdisciplinary Review of Demonic Possession between 1980 and 2023: A Compendium of Scientific Cases. *Journal of Scientific Exploration*, **37**, 633–664.

Espedal, G. (2021) 'Hope to See the Soul': The Relationship between Spirituality and Hope. *Journal of Religion and Health*, **60**, 2770–2783.

Esquirol, J. E. D. (1845) *Mental Maladies: A Treatise on Insanity*: New York: Hafner.

Evans, J. (2024) Where Is the Most Religious Place in the World? Pew Research Center, 9 August. www.pewresearch.org/short-reads/2024/08/09/where-is-the-most-religious-place-in-the-world/.

Evans, J., Lesage, K., Corichi, M. (2025a) *Many Religious 'Nones' around the World Hold Spiritual Beliefs*. Washington, DC: Pew Research Center.

Evans, J., Lesage, K., Miner, W., Starr, K. J., Corichi, M. (2025b) *Believing in Spirits and Life after Death Is Common around the World*. Washington, DC: Pew Research Center.

Exline, J. J. & Rose, E. D. (2013) Religious and Spiritual Struggles. In Paloutzian, R. F. & Park, C. L. (Eds.), *Handbook of the Psychology of Religion and Spirituality*. New York: Guilford Press, 380–398.

Exline, J. J., Pargament, K. I., Grubbs, J. B. & Yali, A. M. (2014) The Religious and Spiritual Struggles Scale: Development and Initial Validation. *Psychology of Religion and Spirituality*, **6**, 208–222.

Exline, J. J., Pargament, K. I., Wilt, J. A. & Harriott, V. A. (2021) Mental Illness, Normal Psychological Processes, or Attacks by the Devil? Three Lenses to Frame Demonic Struggles in Therapy. *Spirituality in Clinical Practice*, **8**, 215–228.

Fagg, D. (2023) Proselytising and Pastoral Care: Chaplains in Australian Government Schools. *Journal of Beliefs and Values*, **45**, 439–453.

Fernandez, F. & Francis, J. (2022) Interpersonal Friendship: A Prerequisite to Mystical Contemplation, According to St Teresa of Avila. *Journal for the Study of Religion*, **35**, 1–19.

Fernyhough, C. (2016) *The Voices Within: The History and Science of How We Talk to Ourselves*. London: Profile.

Fitzgerald, D. & Callard, F. (2016) Entangling the Medical Humanities. In Whitehead, A., Woods, A., Atkinson, S., Macnaughton, J. & Richards, J. (Eds.), *The Edinburgh Companion to the Critical Medical Humanities*. Edinburgh: Edinburgh University Press, 35–49.

Flannelly, K. J., Galek, K., Ellison, C. G. & Koenig, H. G. (2010) Beliefs about God, Psychiatric Symptoms, and Evolutionary Psychiatry. *Journal of Religion and Health*, **49**, 246–261.

Fletcher, J. (Ed.) (2019) *Chaplaincy and Spiritual Care in Mental Health Settings*. London: Jessica Kingsley.

Fonteijn, W. A. (2020) The Impact of Kundalini Awakening on Personal Life and Psychotherapeutic Practice. *Journal of Clinical Case Studies, Reviews and Reports*, **2**, 1–3.

Forrester-Jones, R., Dietzfelbinger, L., Stedman, D. & Richmond, P. (2018) Including the 'Spiritual' within Mental Health Care in the UK, from the Experiences of People with Mental Health Problems. *Journal of Religion and Health*, **57**, 384–407.

Francis, L. J. & Robbins, M. (2008) Psychological Type and Prayer Preferences: A Study among Anglican Clergy in the United Kingdom. *Mental Health, Religion and Culture*, **11**, 67–84.

Francis, L. J., Cook, C. C. H. & McKenna, U. (2025) Psychological Temperament, Spirituality, and Augustinian Prayer: An Empirical Enquiry. *Journal of Spiritual Formation and Soul Care*, **18**, 99–109.

Fraser, G. A. (1993) Exorcism Rituals: Effects on Multiple Personality Disorder Patients. *Dissociation*, **VI**, 239–244.

Freud, S. (1975) *The Pelican Freud Library, Vol. 5: The Psychopathology of Everyday Life*. Ed. Richards, A. (based on the trans. by Strachey, J.). Harmondsworth: Pelican.

Freud, S. (1985a) *The Pelican Freud Library, Vol. 12: Civilization, Society and Religion – Group Psychology, Civilization and Its Discontents and Other Works*. Eds. Strachey, J. & Dickson, A. Harmondsworth: Pelican.

Freud, S. (1985b) *The Pelican Freud Library, Vol. 14: Art and Literature*. Ed. Dickson, A. Harmondsworth: Pelican.

Freud, S. (2012) *The Future of an Illusion*. Ed. Dufresne, T. & Trans. Richter, G. C. Ontario: Broadview.

Froese, P., Bonhag, R., Uecker, J., Andersson, M. & Upenieks, L. (2024) Prayer and Mental Well-Being in the United States: An Overview of Original and Comprehensive Prayer Data. *Journal of Religion and Health*, **63**, 4745–4772.

Gadit, A. A. (2009) Myth of Reincarnation: A Challenge for Mental Health Profession. *Journal of Medical Ethics*, **35**, 91.

Galanter, M., Larson, D. & Rubenstone, E. (1991) Christian Psychiatry: The Impact of Evangelical Belief on Clinical Practice. *American Journal of Psychiatry*, **148**, 90–95.

Galanter, M., Josipovic, Z., Dermatis, H., Weber, J. & Millard, M. A. (2017) An Initial fMRI Study on Neural Correlates of Prayer in Members of Alcoholics Anonymous. *American Journal of Drug and Alcohol Abuse*, **43**, 44–54.

Galanter, M., White, W. L., Ziegler, P. P. & Hunter, B. (2020) An Empirical Study on the Construct of 'God' in the Twelve Step Process. *American Journal of Drug and Alcohol Abuse*, **46**, 731–738.

Galbadage, T., Peterson, B. M., Wang, D. C., Wang, J. S. & Gunasekera, R. S. (2020) Biopsychosocial and Spiritual Implications of Patients with Covid-19 Dying in Isolation. *Frontiers in Psychology*, **11**, 588623.

Galen, L. W. & Kloet, J. D. (2010) Mental Well-Being in the Religious and the Non-religious: Evidence for a Curvilinear Relationship. *Mental Health, Religion and Culture*, **14**, 673–689.

Gallagher, R. (2022) *Demonic Foes*. New York: HarperOne.

Garssen, B., Visser, A. & Pool, G. (2020) Does Spirituality or Religion Positively Affect Mental Health? Meta-analysis of Longitudinal Studies. *International Journal for the Psychology of Religion*, **31**, 4–20.

Gaw, A. C., Ding, Q.-Z., Levine, R. E. & Gaw, H.-F. (1998) The Clinical Characteristics of Possession Disorder among 20 Chinese Patients in the Hebei Province of China. *Psychiatric Services*, **49**, 360–365.

Geertz, C. (1993) Religion as a Cultural System. In Geertz, C. (Ed.), *The Interpretation of Cultures: Selected Essays*. New York: Fontana, 87–125.

General Medical Council (2013) *Personal Beliefs and Medical Practice*. London: General Medical Council.

Gethin, R. (2011) On Some Definitions of Mindfulness. *Contemporary Buddhism*, **12**, 263–279.

Gingrich, H. J. D. (2006) Trauma and Dissociation in the Philippines. *Journal of Trauma Practice*, **4**, 245–269.

Glannon, W. (2020) Mind-Brain Dualism in Psychiatry: Ethical Implications. *Frontiers in Psychiatry*, **11**, 85.

Goff, D. C., Brotman, A. W., Kindlon, D., Waites, M. & Amico, E. (1991) The Delusion of Possession in Chronically Psychotic Patients. *Journal of Nervous and Mental Disease*, **179**, 567–571.

Goh, R. Z., Phillips, I. B. & Firestone, C. (2023) The Perception of Silence. *Proceedings of the National Academy of Sciences of the United States of America*, **120**, e2301463120.

Goldberg, S. B., Tucker, R. P., Greene, P. A., Davidson, R. J., Wampold, B. E.,

Kearney, D. J. & Simpson, T. L. (2018) Mindfulness-Based Interventions for Psychiatric Disorders: A Systematic Review and Meta-analysis. *Clinical Psychology Review*, **59**, 52–60.

Gontijo, D. F., Silva, D. M. R. & Damásio, B. F. (2022) Religiosity/Spirituality and Mental Health: Evidence of Curvilinear Relationships in a Sample of Religious People, Spirituals, Atheists, and Agnostics. *Archive for the Psychology of Religion*, **44**, 69–90.

Gould, S. J. (1999) *Rock of Ages: Science and Religion in the Fullness of Life*. New York: Ballantine.

Gray, A. J. (2011) Worldviews. *International Psychiatry*, **8**, 58–60.

Greenfield, S. M. (2004) Treating the Sick with a Morality Play: The Kardecist-Spiritist Disobsession in Brazil. *Social Analysis*, **48**, 174–194.

Greenway, A. P., Milne, L. C. & Clarke, V. (2003) Personality Variables, Self-Esteem and Depression and an Individual's Perception of God. *Mental Health, Religion and Culture*, **6**, 45–58.

Groves, P. & Farmer, R. (1994) Buddhism and Addictions. *Addiction Research*, **2**, 183–194.

Guze, S. B. (1989) Biological Psychiatry: Is There Any Other Kind? *Psychological Medicine*, **19**, 315–23.

Habermas, J. (2008) Notes on Post-Secular Society. *New Perspectives Quarterly*, **25**, 17–29.

Haeri, N. (2013) The Private Performance of Salat Prayers: Repetition, Time, and Meaning. *Anthropological Quarterly*, **86**, 5–34.

Hahn, J. L. (2020) God as We Understood Him. *Implicit Religion*, **22**, 101–121.

Hale, A. S. & Pinninti, N. R. (1994) Exorcism-Resistant Ghost Possession Treated with Clopenthixol. *British Journal of Psychiatry*, **165**, 386–388.

Hammer, O. (2004) *Claiming Knowledge: Strategies of Epistemology from Theosophy to the New Age*. Leiden: Brill.

Haraldsson, E. (2013) Popular Psychology, Belief in Life after Death and Reincarnation in the Nordic Countries, Western and Eastern Europe. *Nordic Psychology*, **58**, 171–180.

Harris, J. I., Erbes, C. R., Engdahl, B. E., Tedeschi, R. G., Olson, R. H., Winskowski, A. M. M. & McMahill, J. (2010) Coping Functions of Prayer and Posttraumatic Growth. *International Journal for the Psychology of Religion*, **20**, 26–38.

Hart, L. C., Poston, J. M. & Wang, D. C. (2024) God Image as a Moderator of God Concept's Relation to Shame, Depression, and Existential Well-Being among Seminarians. *Psychology of Religion and Spirituality*, **16**, 240–250.

Hartog, K. & Gow, K. M. (2005) Religious Attributions Pertaining to the Causes and Cures of Mental Illness. *Mental Health, Religion and Culture*, **8**, 263–276.

Hastings, S. (2020) *Wrestling with My Thoughts: A Doctor with Mental Illness Discovers Strength*. London: IVP.

Hayward, R. D., Krause, N., Ironson, G., Hill, P. C., Emmons, R. (2016) Health and Well-Being among the Non-religious: Atheists, Agnostics, and No Preference Compared with Religious Group Members. *Journal of Religion and Health*, **55**(3), 1024–1037.

Hecker, T., Braitmayer, L. & Van Duijl, M. (2015) Global Mental Health and Trauma Exposure: The Current Evidence for the Relationship between Traumatic Experiences and Spirit Possession. *European Journal of Psychotraumatology*, **6**, 29126.

Hecker, T., Barnewitz, E., Stenmark, H. & Iversen, V. (2016) Pathological Spirit Possession as a Cultural Interpretation of Trauma-Related Symptoms. *Psychological Trauma*, **8**, 468–476.

Heiler, F. (1932) *Prayer: A Study in the History and Psychology of Religion*. New York: Oxford University Press.

Heinonen, E. & Nissen-Lie, H. A. (2020) The Professional and Personal Characteristics of Effective Psychotherapists: A Systematic Review. *Psychotherapy Research*, **30**, 417–432.

Hernandez, S. E., Barros-Loscertales, A., Xiao, Y., Gonzalez-Mora, J. L. & Rubia, K.

(2018) Gray Matter and Functional Connectivity in Anterior Cingulate Cortex Are Associated with the State of Mental Silence during Sahaja Yoga Meditation. *Neuroscience*, **371**, 395–406.

Heyd, M. (1995) *'Be Sober and Reasonable': The Critique of Enthusiasm in the Seventeenth and Early Eighteenth Centuries*. Leiden: Brill.

Hiatt, J. F. (1986) Spirituality, Medicine, and Healing. *Southern Medical Journal*, **79**, 736–743.

Hinton, D. E. & Lewis-Fernandez, R. (2010) Idioms of Distress among Trauma Survivors: Subtypes and Clinical Utility. *Culture, Medicine, and Psychiatry*, **34**, 209–218.

Hirshberg, M. J., Goldberg, S. B., Rosenkranz, M. & Davidson, R. J. (2022) Prevalence of Harm in Mindfulness-Based Stress Reduction. *Psychological Medicine*, **52**, 1080–1088.

Holmes, J. (2024) *The Spirit of Psychotherapy: A Hidden Dimension*. Bicester: Karnac.

Hoover, J. (2018) Can Christians Practice Mindfulness without Compromising Their Convictions? *Journal of Psychology and Christianity*, **37**, 247–255.

Huang Harris, J., Chennankara, S., Thielman, S. & Peteet, J. R. (2024) Treating Evangelical Christians: Challenges and Opportunities. *Psychiatric Services*, **75**, 1049–1052.

Huguelet, P. & Koenig, H. G. (Eds.) (2009) *Religion and Spirituality in Psychiatry*. Cambridge: Cambridge University Press.

Humpston, C. S. & Broome, M. R. (2015) The Spectra of Soundless Voices and Audible Thoughts: Towards an Integrative Model of Auditory Verbal Hallucinations and Thought Insertion. *Review of Philosophy and Psychology*, **7**(3), 611–629.

Husain, A. & Hodge, D. R. (2016) Islamically Modified Cognitive Behavioral Therapy: Enhancing Outcomes by Increasing the Cultural Congruence of Cognitive Behavioral Therapy Self-Statements. *International Social Work*, **59**, 393–405.

Huxley, A. (1971) *The Devils of Loudun*. Harmondsworth: Penguin.

Idler, E., Levin, J., Vanderweele, T. J. & Khan, A. (2019) Partnerships between Public Health Agencies and Faith Communities. *American Journal of Public Health*, **109**, 346–347.

Igberase, O. & Okogbenin, E. (2017) Beliefs about the Cause of Schizophrenia among Caregivers in Midwestern Nigeria. *Mental Illness*, **9**, 6983.

Iida, J. (1989) The Current Situation in Regard to the Delusion of Possession in Japan. *Japanese Journal of Psychiatry*, **43**, 19–27.

Ijaz, S., Khalily, M. T. & Ahmad, I. (2017) Mindfulness in Salah Prayer and Its Association with Mental Health. *Journal of Religion and Health*, **56**, 2297–2307.

Illich, I. D. (1973) *Celebration of Awareness: A Call for Institutional Revolution*. Harmondsworth: Penguin.

Islam, F. & Campbell, R. A. (2014) 'Satan Has Afflicted Me!' Jinn-Possession and Mental Illness in the Qur'an. *Journal of Religion and Health*, **53**, 229–243.

Isobel, S., Gladstone, B., Goodyear, M., Furness, T. & Foster, K. (2021) A Qualitative Inquiry into Psychiatrists' Perspectives on the Relationship of Psychological Trauma to Mental Illness and Treatment: Implications for Trauma-Informed Care. *Journal of Mental Health*, **30**, 667–673.

Jackson, M. (2004) The Prose of Suffering and the Practice of Silence. *Spiritus: A Journal of Christian Spirituality*, **4**, 44–59.

Jackson, P. & Cook, C. C. H. (2005) Introduction of a Spirituality Group in a Community Service for People with Drinking Problems. *Journal of Substance Use*, **10**, 375–383.

Jafari, M. F. (1993) Counseling Values and Objectives: A Comparison of Western and Islamic Perspectives. *American Journal of Islamic Social Studies*, **10**, 326–339.

Jaffé, A., Winston, R. & Winston, C. (Eds.) (1963) *C.G. Jung: Memories, Dreams, Reflections*. London: Collins.

Janse Van Rensburg, A. B. R. (2014) South African Society of Psychiatrists Guidelines for the Integration of Spirituality in the Approach to Psychiatric Practice. *South African Journal of Psychiatry*, **20**, 133–139.

Jennings, J. L. (2024) Engaging with the Unknown: How Judaism Enabled Freud's

Psychological Discoveries. *Journal of the History of the Behavioral Sciences*, **60**, e22293.

Jeppsen, B., Winkeljohn Black, S., Pössel, P. & Rosmarin, D. H. (2022) Does Closeness to God Mediate the Relationship between Prayer and Mental Health in Christian, Jewish, and Muslim Samples? *Mental Health, Religion and Culture*, **25**, 99–112.

Jonker, H. S., Eurelings-Bontekoe, E. H. M., Zock, H. & Jonker, E. (2008) Development and Validation of the Dutch Questionnaire God Image: Effects of Mental Health and Religious Culture. *Mental Health, Religion and Culture*, **11**, 501–515.

Jung, C. G. (1986) *Collected Works, Vol. 11: Psychology and Religion – West and East*. Eds. & Trans. Adler, G. & Hull, R. F. C. Princeton, NJ: Princeton University Press.

Kabat-Zinn, J. (2020) *Full Catastrophe Living: How to Cope with Stress, Pain and Illness Using Mindfulness Meditation*. London: Piatkus.

Kang, C. (2010) Hinduism and Mental Health: Engaging British Hindus. *Mental Health, Religion and Culture*, **13**, 587–593.

Katz, M. H. (2013) *Prayer in Islamic Thought and Practice*. Cambridge: Cambridge University Press.

Kavanaugh, K. & Rodriguez, O. (1985) *The Collected Works of St Teresa of Avila*. Washington, DC: Institute of Carmelite Studies.

Kavanaugh, K. & Rodriguez, O. (1991) *The Collected Works of St John of the Cross*. Washington, DC: Institute of Carmelite Studies.

Kelly, E. (2012) The Development of Healthcare Chaplaincy. *The Expository Times*, **123**, 469–478.

Kenny, C. (2021) Encountering Religious and Spiritual Silences. In Dimitrijević, A. & Buchholz, M. B. (Eds.), *Silence and Silencing in Psychoanalysis*. London: Routledge, 26–40.

Kerr, D. A. (1999) Christian Understandings of Proselytism. *International Bulletin of Missionary Research*, **23**, 8–14.

Khaksari, Z. & Khosravi, Z. (2011) Positive and Negative Conception of God and Its Relationship with Student's Self-Esteem and Mental Health. *Journal of Life Sciences and Biomedicine*, **2**, 62–68.

Khalifa, N. & Hardie, T. (2005) Possession and Jinn. *Journal of the Royal Society of Medicine*, **98**, 351–353.

Kharitidi, O. (1996) *Entering the Circle: Ancient Secrets of Siberian Wisdom Discovered by a Russian Psychiatrist*. London: Thorsons.

Kharitidi, O. (2001) *Master of Lucid Dreams*. Charlottesville, VA: Hampton Roads.

Kierkegaard, S. (1961) *Purity of Heart Is to Will One Thing*. London: Fontana.

Kinghorn, W. A. (2016) American Christian Engagement with Mental Health and Mental Illness. *Psychiatric Services*, **67**, 107–110.

Kirmayer, L. J. & Crafa, D. (2014) What Kind of Science for Psychiatry? *Frontiers in Human Neuroscience*, **8**, article 435.

Kirmayer, L. J. & Gold, I. (2011) Re-socializing Psychiatry: Critical Neuroscience and the Limits of Reductionism. In Choudhury, S. & Slaby, J. (Eds.), *Critical Neuroscience: A Handbook of the Social and Cultural Contexts of Neuroscience*. Oxford: Wiley-Blackwell, 307–330.

Klemm, W. R. (2019) Whither Neurotheology? *Religions*, **10**, article 634.

Knott, K. (2016) *Hinduism: A Very Short Introduction*. Oxford: Oxford University Press.

Koenig, H. G. (2008a) Concerns about Measuring 'Spirituality' in Research. *Journal of Nervous and Mental Disease*, **196**, 349–355.

Koenig, H. G. (2008b) Religion and Mental Health: What Should Psychiatrists Do? *Psychiatric Bulletin*, **32**, 201–203.

Koenig, H. G. (2013) *Spirituality in Patient Care: Why, How, When, and What*. West Conshohocken, PA: Templeton.

Koenig, H. G. (2014) The Spiritual Care Team: Enabling the Practice of Whole Person Medicine. *Religions*, **5**, 1161–1174.

Koenig, H. G. (2018) *Religion and Mental Health: Research and Clinical Applications*. London: Academic Press.

Koenig, H. G. (2023) Person-Centered Mindfulness: A Culturally and Spiritually Sensitive Approach to Clinical Practice.

Journal of Religion and Health, **62**, 1884–1896.

Koenig, H. G. & Larson, D. B. (2001) Religion and Mental Health: Evidence for an Association. *International Review of Psychiatry*, **13**, 67–78.

Koenig, H. G., Pearce, M. J., Nelson, B., Shaw, S. F., Robins, C. J., Daher, N. S., Cohen, H. J., Berk, L. S., Bellinger, D. L., Pargament, K. I., Rosmarin, D. H., Vasegh, S., Kristeller, J., Juthani, N., Nies, D. & King, M. B. (2015) Religious vs Conventional Cognitive Behavioral Therapy for Major Depression in Persons with Chronic Medical Illness: A Pilot Randomized Trial. *Journal of Nervous and Mental Disease*, **203**, 243–251.

Koenig, H. G., Hill, T. D., Pirutinsky, S. & Rosmarin, D. H. (2020a) Commentary on 'Does Spirituality or Religion Positively Affect Mental Health?' *International Journal for the Psychology of Religion*, **31**, 27–44.

Koenig, H. G., Peteet, J. R. & Vanderweele, T. J. (2020b) Religion and Psychiatry: Clinical Applications. *BJPsych Advances*, **26**, 273–281.

Koenig, H. G., Vanderweele, T. J. & Peteet, J. R. (2024) *Handbook of Religion and Health*. Oxford: Oxford University Press.

Koohsar, A. A. H. & Bonab, B. G. (2011a) Relation between Quality of Image of God and Mental Health in College Students. *Procedia – Social and Behavioral Sciences*, **29**, 247–251.

Koohsar, A. A. H. & Bonab, B. G. (2011b) Relation between Quality of Image of God with Anxiety and Depression in College Students. *Procedia – Social and Behavioral Sciences*, **29**, 252–256.

Kugelmass, H. & Garcia, A. (2015) Mental Disorder among Nonreligious Adolescents. *Mental Health, Religion and Culture*, **18**, 368–379.

Kuhn, C. C. (1988) A Spiritual Inventory of the Medically Ill Patient. *Psychiatric Medicine*, **6**, 87–100.

Kurhade, C., Jagannathan, A., Varambally, S. & Shivanna, S. (2022) Religion-Based Interventions for Mental Health Disorders: A Systematic Review. *Journal of Applied Consciousness Studies*, **10**, 20–33.

Kurtz, E. (1991) *Not-God: A History of Alcoholics Anonymous*. Center City, MN: Hazelden.

Ladany, N., Hill, C. E., Thompson, B. J. & O'Brien, K. M. (2006) Therapist Perspectives on Using Silence in Therapy: A Qualitative Study. *Counselling and Psychotherapy Research*, **4**, 80–89.

Ladd, K. L., Vreugdenhil, S. L., Ladd, M. L. & Cook, C. A. (2012) Interpersonal Conversations and Prayers: Differences of Content and Attachment Functions. *Journal of Communication and Religion*, **35**, 295–314.

Ladd, K. L., Cook, C. A., Foreman, K. M. & Ritter, E. A. (2015) Neuroimaging of Prayer: Questions of Validity. *Psychology of Religion and Spirituality*, **7**, 100–108.

Ladd, K. L., Ladd, M. L. & Sahai, N. (2018) Conceptualizing 'Prayer' for an East–West Dialogue and Beyond. *Psychological Studies*, **23**, 163–171.

Lake, F. (1966) *Clinical Theology*. London: Darton, Longman & Todd.

Lamothe, R. (2003) Freud, Religion, and the Presence of Projective Identification. *Psychoanalytic Psychology*, **20**, 287–302.

Lane, R. C., Koetting, M. G. & Bishop, J. (2002) Silence as Communication in Dynamic Psychotherapy. *Clinical Psychology Review*, **22**, 1091–1104.

Leach, M. M., Piedmont, R. L. & Monteiro, D. (2001) Images of God among Christians, Hindus and Muslims in India. *Research in the Social Scientific Study of Religion*, **12**, 207–225.

Leamy, M., Bird, V., Le Boutillier, C., Williams, J. & Slade, M. (2011) Conceptual Framework for Personal Recovery in Mental Health: Systematic Review and Narrative Synthesis. *British Journal of Psychiatry*, **199**, 445–452.

Leff, J. (1975) 'Exotic' Treatments and Western Psychiatry. *Psychological Medicine*, **5**, 125–128.

Levin, J., Bradshaw, M., Johnson, B. R. & Stark, R. (2022) Are Religious 'Nones' Really Not Religious? Revisiting Glenn, Three

Decades Later. *Interdisciplinary Journal of Research on Religion*, **17**, 1–28.

Levitt, C. & Turgeon, A. (2009) Sigmund Freud's Intensive Reading of Ludwig Feuerbach. *Canadian Journal of Psychoanalysis*, **17**, 14–35.

Levitt, H. M. & Morrill, Z. (2023) Silences in Psychotherapy: An Integrative Meta-analytic Research Review. *Psychotherapy (Chicago, IL)*, **60**, 320–341.

Lewis, A. (1951) Henry Maudsley: His Work and Influence. *Journal of Mental Science*, **97**, 259–277.

Lewis, I. M. (1975) *Ecstatic Religion: An Anthropological Study of Spirit Possession and Shamanism*. Harmondsworth: Penguin.

Lhermitte, J. (1963) *Diabolical Possession, True and False*. London: Burns & Oates.

Lilley, A., Moss, R., Van De Kasteele, P. & Hughes, G. (2016) Clinical Theology Revisited. *Contact*, **122**, 23–30.

Lim, A., Hoek, H. W., Ghane, S., Deen, M. & Blom, J. D. (2018) The Attribution of Mental Health Problems to Jinn: An Explorative Study in a Transcultural Psychiatric Outpatient Clinic. *Frontiers in Psychiatry*, **9**, 89.

Lindbeck, G. A. (2009) *The Nature of Doctrine: Religion and Theology in a Postliberal Age*. Louisville, KY: Westminster John Knox Press.

Littlewood, R. (2004) Possession States. *Psychiatry*, **3**, 8–10.

Long, K. N. G., Symons, X., Vanderweele, T. J., Balboni, T. A., Rosmarin, D. H., Puchalski, C., Cutts, T., Gunderson, G. R., Idler, E., Oman, D., Balboni, M. J., Tuach, L. S. & Koh, H. K. (2024) Spirituality as a Determinant of Health: Emerging Policies, Practices, and Systems. *Health Affairs (Millwood)*, **43**, 783–790.

Lowe, G. B., Wang, D. C. & Chin, E. G. (2022) Experiential Avoidance Mediates the Relationship between Prayer Type and Mental Health before and through the Covid-19 Pandemic. *Religions*, **13**, 652.

Lucchetti, G., Aguiar, P. R., Braghetta, C. C., Vallada, C. P., Moreira-Almeida, A. & Vallada, H. (2012) Spiritist Psychiatric Hospitals in Brazil: Integration of Conventional Psychiatric Treatment and Spiritual Complementary Therapy. *Culture, Medicine, and Psychiatry*, **36**, 124–35.

Luhrmann, T. M. (2012) *When God Talks Back*. New York: Knopf.

Luhrmann, T. M. (2020) *How God Becomes Real: Kindling the Presence of Invisible Others*. Princeton, NJ: Princeton University Press.

Lupfer, M. B., Tolliver, D. & Jackson, M. (1996) Explaining Life-Altering Occurrences: A Test of the 'God-of-the-Gaps' Hypothesis. *Journal for the Scientific Study of Religion*, **35**, 379–391.

Lysaught, M. T. (2004) Respect: Or, How Respect for Persons Became Respect for Autonomy. *Journal of Medicine and Philosophy*, **29**, 665–680.

Mace, C. (2008) *Mindfulness and Mental Health*. London: Routledge.

MacIntyre, A. (1966) Visions. In Flew, A. & MacIntyre, A. (Eds.), *New Essays in Philosophical Theology*. London: SCM, 254–260.

MacKenna, C. (2002) Self Images and God Images. *British Journal of Psychotherapy*, **18**, 325–338.

Macmin, L. & Foskett, J. (2004) 'Don't Be Afraid to Tell': The Spiritual and Religious Experience of Mental Health Service Users in Somerset. *Mental Health, Religion and Culture*, **7**, 23–40.

Mahmoodabad, S. S. M., Tabei, S. Z., Nami, M., Fallahzadeh, H., Jahromi, B. N., Shayan, A. & Forouhari, S. (2016) Extrinsic or Intrinsic Religious Orientation May Have an Impact on Mental Health. *Research Journal of Medical Sciences*, **10**, 232–236.

Main, R. (2006) Religion. In Papadopoulos, R. (Ed.), *The Handbook of Jungian Psychology: Theory, Practice and Applications*. London: Routledge, 296–323.

Maniam, T. (1987) Exorcism and Psychiatric Illness: Two Case Reports. *Medical Journal of Malaysia*, **42**, 317–319.

Mars, R. B., Neubert, F. X., Noonan, M. P., Sallet, J., Toni, I. & Rushworth, M. F. (2012) On the Relationship between the 'Default Mode Network' and the 'Social Brain'. *Frontiers in Human Neuroscience*, **6**, 189.

Martin, D. (2005) *On Secularization: Towards a Revised General Theory*. Aldershot: Ashgate.

Martínez De Pisón, R. (2022) Religion, Spirituality and Mental Health: The Role of Guilt and Shame. *Journal of Spirituality in Mental Health*, **25**, 261–276.

Mason, M. F., Norton, M. I., Van Horn, J. D., Wegner, D. M., Grafton, S. T. & Macrae, N. (2007) Wandering Minds: The Default Network and Stimulus-Independent Thought. *Science*, **315**, 393–395.

Maudsley, H. ([1895] 1979) *The Pathology of Mind*. London: Friedmann.

May, G. G. (1982) *Will and Spirit: A Contemplative Psychology*. San Francisco, CA: HarperCollins.

McCall, W. V. (2006) Psychiatry and Psychology in the Writings of L. Ron Hubbard. *Journal of Religion and Health*, **46**, 437–447.

McCarthy, M. (2014) US Doctors Are Judged More on Bedside Manner Than Effectiveness of Care, Survey Finds. *British Medical Journal*, **349**, g4864.

McFadyen, A. (2000) *Bound to Sin: Abuse, Holocaust and the Christian Doctrine of Sin*. Cambridge: Cambridge University Press.

McGilchrist, I. (2011) Paying Attention to the Bipartite Brain. *The Lancet*, **377**, 1068–1069.

McGilchrist, I. (2019) Cerebral Lateralization and Religion: A Phenomenological Approach. *Religion, Brain and Behavior*, **9**, 319–339.

McGrath, A. (2009) *A Fine-Tuned Universe: The Quest for God in Science and Theology*. Louisville, KY: Westminster John Knox Press.

McKee, D. D. & Chappel, J. N. (1992) Spirituality and Medical Practice. *Journal of Family Practice*, **35**, 205–208.

McLeish, T. (2014) *Faith and Wisdom in Science*. Oxford: Oxford University Press.

Menegatti-Chequini, M. C., Loch, A. A., Leao, F. C., Peres, M. F. P. & Vallada, H. (2020) Patterns of Religiosity and Spirituality of Psychiatrists in Brazil and the Implications for Clinical Practice: A Latent Profile Analysis. *BMC (BioMed Central) Psychiatry*, **20**, 546.

Meng, H. & Freud, E. L. (Eds.) (1963) *Psychoanalysis and Faith: The Letters of Sigmund Freud and Oskar Pfister*. London: Hogarth Press.

Mental Health Foundation (2002) *Taken Seriously: The Somerset Spirituality Project*. London: Mental Health Foundation.

Mercadante, L. (2014) *Belief without Borders: Inside the Minds of the Spiritual but Not Religious*. Oxford: Oxford University Press.

Mercadante, L. (2020) Spiritual Struggles of Nones and 'Spiritual but Not Religious' (SBNRs). *Religions*, **11**(10), 513.

Merton, T. (1969) *The Climate of Monastic Prayer*. Kalamazoo, MI: Cistercian Publications.

Michael, C. P. & Norrisey, M. C. (1984) *Prayer and Temperament*. Charlottesville, VA: Open Door.

Milner, K., Crawford, P., Edgley, A., Hare-Duke, L. & Slade, M. (2020) The Experiences of Spirituality among Adults with Mental Health Difficulties: A Qualitative Systematic Review. *Epidemiology and Psychiatric Sciences*, **29**, e34.

Milner, M. (1950) *On Not Being Able to Paint*. London: Routledge.

Moore, J. T. & Leach, M. M. (2016) Dogmatism and Mental Health: A Comparison of the Religious and Secular. *Psychology of Religion and Spirituality*, **8**, 54–64.

Moreira-Almeida, A. (2009) Differentiating Spiritual from Psychotic Experiences. *British Journal of Psychiatry*, **195**, 370–371.

Moreira-Almeida, A. & Lotufo Neto, F. (2005) Spiritist Views of Mental Disorders in Brazil. *Transcultural Psychiatry*, **42**, 570–595.

Moreira-Almeida, A., Sharma, A., Van Rensburg, B. J., Verhagen, P. J. & Cook, C. C. H. (2016) WPA Position Statement on Spirituality and Religion in Psychiatry. *World Psychiatry*, **15**, 87–88.

Moreira-Almeida, A., Mosqueiro, B. P. & Bhugra, D. (Eds.) (2021) *Spirituality and Mental Health across Cultures*. Oxford: Oxford University Press.

Moreira-Almeida, A., De Abreu Costa, M. & Coelho, H. S. (2022) *Science of Life after Death*. Cham: Springer.

Mosqueiro, B. P., Costa, M. A., Caribe, A. C., Oliveira e Oliveira, F. H. A., Pizutti, L., Zimpel, R. R., Baldacara, L., da Silva, A. G. & Moreira-Almeida, A. (2023) Brazilian Psychiatric Association Guidelines on the Integration of Spirituality into Mental Health Clinical Practice: Part 1. Spiritual History and Differential Diagnosis. *Brazilian Journal of Psychiatry*, **45**(6), 506–517.

Murphy, M. A. (2010) *Voices in the Rain: Meaning in Psychosis*. Eugene, OR: WIPF & Stock.

Murphy, M. A. (2024) *The Compassionate Psychiatrist: Redefining Mental Healthcare*. Eugene, OR: Resource Publications.

Neil, P. (2015) Ordinary Sacramental Theology in Rural Wales. *Rural Theology*, **11**, 28–38.

Newberg, A. B. (2010) *Principles of Neurotheology*. Farnham: Ashgate.

Nguyen, H. T., Yamada, A. M. & Dinh, T. Q. (2012) Religious Leaders' Assessment and Attribution of the Causes of Mental Illness: An In-Depth Exploration of Vietnamese American Buddhist Leaders. *Mental Health, Religion and Culture*, **15**, 511–527.

Nichter, M. (1981) Idioms of Distress: Alternatives in the Expression of Psychosocial Distress: A Case Study from South India. *Culture, Medicine and Psychiatry*, **5**, 379–408.

Nie, F. & Olson, D. V. A. (2016) Demonic Influence: The Negative Mental Health Effects of Belief in Demons. *Journal for the Scientific Study of Religion*, **55**, 498–515.

Noll, R. (1985) Mental Imagery Cultivation as a Cultural Phenomenon: The Role of Visions in Shamanism. *Current Anthropology*, **26**, 443–459.

Noorani, T. (2022) Conspiration in the Archive: Sense-Making and the Research Interview Methodology. In Woods, A., Alderson-Day, B. & Fernyhough, C. (Eds.), *Voices in Psychosis: Interdisciplinary Perspectives*. Oxford: Oxford University Press, 101–107.

Norcross, J. C., Koocher, G. P. & Garofalo, A. (2006) Discredited Psychological Treatments and Tests: A Delphi Poll. *Professional Psychology: Research and Practice*, **37**, 515–522.

Northcott, M. S. & Berry, R. J. (Eds.) (2009) *Theology after Darwin*. Milton Keynes: Paternoster.

Otto, R. (1980) *The Idea of the Holy*. Oxford: Oxford University Press.

Ouwehand, E. (2020) *Mania and Meaning – A Mixed Methods Study into Religious Experiences in People with Bipolar Disorder: Occurrence and Significance*. Groningen: University of Groningen Press.

Ouwehand, E., Wong, K., Boeije, H. & Braam, A. (2014) Revelation, Delusion or Disillusion: Subjective Interpretation of Religious and Spiritual Experiences in Bipolar Disorder. *Mental Health, Religion and Culture*, **17**, 615–628.

Ouwehand, E., Muthert, H., Zock, H., Boeije, H. & Braam, A. (2018) Sweet Delight and Endless Night: A Qualitative Exploration of Ordinary and Extraordinary Religious and Spiritual Experiences in Bipolar Disorder. *International Journal for the Psychology of Religion*, **28**, 31–54.

Oyebode, F. (2018) Editorial: Literature and Psychiatry. *Advances in Psychiatric Treatment*, **8**, 397–398.

Oyebode, F. (2023) *Sims' Symptoms in the Mind*. Amsterdam: Elsevier.

Padmanabhan, D. (2017) From Distress to Disease: A Critique of the Medicalisation of Possession in DSM-5. *Anthropology and Medicine*, **24**, 261–275.

Pantelidou, M. & Demetriades, A. K. (2014) The Enigmatic Figure of Dr Henry Maudsley (1835–1918). *Journal of Medical Biography*, **22**, 180–188.

Pargament, K. I. (2011) *Spiritually Integrated Psychotherapy*. New York: Guilford Press.

Pargament, K. I. & Exline, J. J. (2022) *Working with Spiritual Struggles in Psychotherapy*. New York: Guilford Press.

Pargament, K. I., Kennell, J., Hathaway, W., Grevengoed, N., Newman, J. & Jones, W. (1988) Religion and the Problem-Solving Process: Three Styles of Coping. *Journal for the Scientific Study of Religion*, **27**, 90–104.

Pargament, K. I., Ensing, D. S., Falgout, K., Olsen, H., Reilly, B., Van Haltsma, K. & Warren, R. (1990) God Help Me, (I):

Religious Coping Efforts as Predictors of the Outcomes to Significant Life Events. *American Journal of Community Psychology*, **18**, 793–824.

Pargament, K. I., Smith, B. W., Koenig, H. G. & Perez, L. (1998) Patterns of Positive and Negative Religious Coping with Major Life Stressors. *Journal for the Scientific Study of Religion*, **37**, 710–724.

Pargament, K. I., Koenig, H. G., Tarakeshwar, N. & Hahn, J. (2001) Religious Struggle as a Predictor of Mortality among Medically Ill Elderly Patients: A 2-Year Longitudinal Study. *Archives of Internal Medicine*, **161**, 1881–1885.

Park, C. L. (2021) Intrinsic and Extrinsic Religious Motivation: Retrospect and Prospect. *International Journal for the Psychology of Religion*, **31**, 213–222.

Patel, R., Jong, J., Worthington, E. L. & Lycett, D. (2022) The Development of the Religious Health Interventions in Behavioural Science (RHIBS) Taxonomy: A Scientific Classification of Religious Practices in Health. *Translational Behavioral Medicine*, **12**, 987–1003.

Pattison, S. (2007) Absent Friends in Medical Humanities. *Medical Humanities*, **33**, 65–66.

Pearce, M. J., Koenig, H. G., Robins, C. J., Nelson, B., Shaw, S. F., Cohen, H. J. & King, M. B. (2014) Religiously Integrated Cognitive Behavioral Therapy: A New Method of Treatment for Major Depression in Patients with Chronic Medical Illness. *Psychotherapy (Chicago, IL)*, **52**, 56–66.

Peck, M. S. (2005) *Glimpses of the Devil: A Psychiatrist's Personal Account of Possession, Exorcism and Redemption*. New York: Free Press.

Pehlivanova, M., Janke, M. J., Lee, J. & Tucker, J. B. (2018) Childhood Gender Nonconformity and Children's Past-Life Memories. *International Journal of Sexual Health*, **30**, 380–389.

Pennycook, G., Cheyne, J. A., Seli, P., Koehler, D. J. & Fugelsang, J. A. (2012) Analytic Cognitive Style Predicts Religious and Paranormal Belief. *Cognition*, **123**, 335–346.

Peres, J. F. P. (2012) Should Psychotherapy Consider Reincarnation? *Journal of Nervous and Mental Disease*, **200**, 174–179.

Perez, L. G., Cardenas, C., Blagg, T. & Wong, E. C. (2025) Partnerships between Faith Communities and the Mental Health Sector: A Scoping Review. *Psychiatric Services*, **76**, 61–81.

Perry, M. (1996) *Deliverance*. London: SPCK.

Person-Centred Training and Curriculum (PCTC) Scoping Group and Special Committee on Professional Practice and Ethics (2018) *Person-Centred Care: Implications for Training in Psychiatry*. London: Royal College of Psychiatrists.

Peteet, J. R. (2013) What Is the Place of Clinicians' Religious or Spiritual Commitments in Psychotherapy? A Virtues-Based Perspective. *Journal of Religion and Health*, **53**(4), 1190–1198.

Peteet, J. R., Abou-Allaban, Y., Dell, M. L., Greenberg, W., Lomax, J., Torres, M. & Cowell, V. (2006) *Resource Document on Religious/Spiritual Commitments and Psychiatric Practice*. Washington, DC: American Psychiatric Association.

Peteet, J. R., Rodriguez, V. B., Herschkopf, M. D., McCarthy, A., Betts, J., Romo, S. & Murphy, J. M. (2016) Does a Therapist's World View Matter? *Journal of Religion and Health*, **55**, 1097–1106.

Peters, J. (1989) *Frank Lake: The Man and His Work*. London: Darton, Longman & Todd.

Pew Research Center (2018) *The Age Gap in Religion around the World*. Washington, DC: Pew Research Center.

Pew Research Center (2025) *Decline of Christianity in the US Has Slowed, May Have Leveled Off: Findings from the 2023–2024 Religious Landscape Survey*. Washington, DC: Pew Research Center.

Pfeifer, S. (1994) Belief in Demons and Exorcism in Psychiatric Patients in Switzerland. *British Journal of Medical Psychology*, **67**, 247–258.

Pfeifer, S. (1999) Demonic Attributions in Nondelusional Disorders. *Psychopathology*, **32**, 252–259.

Phillips, J., El-Gabalawi, F., Fallon, B. A., Majeed, S., Merlino, J. P., Nields, J. A.,

Saunders, D. & Norko, M. A. (2020) Religion and Psychiatry in the Age of Neuroscience. *Journal of Nervous and Mental Disease*, **208**, 517–523.

Piedmont, R. L. (1999) Does Spirituality Represent the Sixth Factor of Personality? Spiritual Transcendence and the Five-Factor Model. *Journal of Personality*, **67**, 985–1013.

Pimple, K. D. (1995) Ghosts, Spirits, and Scholars: The Origins of Modern Spiritualism. In Walker, B. (Ed.), *Out of the Ordinary*. Boulder: University Press of Colorado, 75–89.

Pirutinsky, S. (2024) Negative Religious Coping Versus Spiritual Struggles: Moderator or Main Effect? *Journal of Clinical Psychology*, **80**(8), 1780–1796.

Polkinghorne, J. (1998) *Science and Theology: An Introduction*. London: SPCK.

Polkinghorne, J. (2000) *Faith, Science and Understanding*. London: SPCK.

Poloma, M. M. & Pendleton, B. F. (1989) Exploring Types of Prayer and Quality of Life: A Research Note. *Review of Religious Research*, **31**, 46–53.

Poole, R. & Cook, C. C. H. (2011) Praying with a Patient Constitutes a Breach of Professional Boundaries in Psychiatric Practice. *British Journal of Psychiatry*, **199**, 94–98.

Poole, R., Higgo, R., Strong, G., Kennedy, G., Ruben, S., Barnes, R., Lepping, P. & Mitchell, P. (2008) Religion, Psychiatry and Professional Boundaries. *Psychiatric Bulletin*, **32**, 356–357.

Poole, R., Cook, C. C. H., Song, R. & Robinson, C. A. (2024) Psychiatrists' Attitudes to Professional Boundaries Concerning Spirituality and Religion: Mixed-Methods Study. *BJPsych Bulletin*, **48**, 221–225.

Possel, P., Winkeljohn Black, S., Bjerg, A. C., Jeppsen, B. D. & Wooldridge, D. T. (2014) Do Trust-Based Beliefs Mediate the Associations of Frequency of Private Prayer with Mental Health? A Cross-Sectional Study. *Journal of Religion and Health*, **53**, 904–916.

Powell, A. J. & Moseley, P. (2021) When Spirits Speak: Absorption, Attribution, and Identity among Spiritualists Who Report 'Clairaudient' Voice Experiences. *Mental Health, Religion and Culture*, **23**, 841–856.

Powers, P. R. (2004) Interiors, Intentions, and the 'Spirituality' of Islamic Ritual Practice. *Journal of the American Academy of Religion*, **72**, 425–459.

Purdam, K., Afkhami, R., Crockett, A. & Olsen, W. (2010) Religion in the UK: An Overview of Equality Statistics and Evidence Gaps. *Journal of Contemporary Religion*, **22**, 147–168.

Rahman, H. A., Hussin, S. & Ridzwan, Z. (2021a) Diagnosis of Jinn Possession Amongst Patients with Mental Disorders Using Thermal Imaging. *Sains Insani*, **6**, 103–106.

Rahman, M. Z. A., Zulkiply, S. R. I. & Mustapha, A. M. (2021b) The Term Waswas and Obsessive-Compulsive Disorder (OCD) in Islamic Perspectives. *Al Hikmah International Journal of Islamic Studies and Human Sciences*, **4**, 452–469.

Rajski, P. (2003) Finding God in the Silence: Contemplative Prayer and Therapy. *Journal of Religion and Health*, **42**, 181–190.

Ramsey-Lucas, C. (2016) Faith and Mental Health: Creating a Culture of Encounter and Friendship. *Review and Expositor*, **113**, 198–204.

Ray, S. D., Lockman, J. D., Jones, E. J. & Kelly, M. H. (2015) Attributions to God and Satan about Life-Altering Events. *Psychology of Religion and Spirituality*, **7**, 60–69.

Richards, P. S. & Bergin, A. E. (Eds.) (2000) *Handbook of Psychotherapy and Religious Diversity*. Washington, DC: American Psychological Association.

Richardson, P. T. (1996) *Four Spiritualities: Expressions of Self, Expressions of Spirit – A Psychology of Contemporary Spiritual Choice*. Palo Alto, CA: Davies-Black.

Rifai, J. E. (2019) A Contested Concept: The Image of God in Islam. *Proceedings of the National Conference on Undergraduate Research (NCUR) 2019 Kennesaw State University*, 991–998.

Rim, J. I., Ojeda, J. C., Svob, C., Kayser, J., Drews, E., Kim, Y., Tenke, C. E., Skipper, J. & Weissman, M. M. (2019) Current

Understanding of Religion, Spirituality, and Their Neurobiological Correlates. *Harvard Review of Psychiatry*, **27**, 303–316.

Rizzuto, A.-M. (1979) *The Birth of the Living God: A Psychoanalytic Study*. Chicago, IL: University of Chicago Press.

Robbins, M., Francis, L. J. & Edwards, B. (2008) Prayer, Personality and Happiness: A Study among Undergraduate Students in Wales. *Mental Health, Religion and Culture*, **11**, 93–99.

Rose, N. & Abi-Rached, J. M. (2013) *Neuro: The New Brain Sciences and the Management of the Mind*. Princeton, NJ: Princeton University Press.

Rosik, C. H. (1997) When Discernment Fails: The Case for Outcome Studies on Exorcism. *Journal of Psychology and Theology*, **25**, 354–363.

Rosmarin, D. H. (2018) *Spirituality, Religion, and Cognitive-Behavioral Therapy*. New York: Guilford Press.

Rosmarin, D. H., Bigda-Peyton, J. S., Ongur, D., Pargament, K. I. & Bjorgvinsson, T. (2013) Religious Coping among Psychotic Patients: Relevance to Suicidality and Treatment Outcomes. *Psychiatry Research*, **210**, 182–187.

Rosmarin, D. H., Salcone, S., Harper, D. & Forester, B. P. (2019) Spiritual Psychotherapy for Inpatient, Residential, and Intensive Treatment. *American Journal of Psychotherapy*, **72**, 75–83.

Ross, A. (2022) *Sigmund Freud: A Reference Guide to His Life and Works*. Lanham, MD: Rowman & Littlefield.

Ross, C. A. (2011) Possession Experiences in Dissociative Identity Disorder: A Preliminary Study. *Journal of Trauma Dissociation*, **12**, 393–400.

Ross, L., Grimwade, L. & Eagger, S. (2022) Spiritual Assessment. In Cook, C. C. H. & Powell, A. (Eds.), *Spirituality and Psychiatry*, 2nd ed. Cambridge: Cambridge University Press, 23–48.

Ross, M. W. & Stålström, O. W. (1979) Exorcism as Psychiatric Treatment: A Homosexual Case Study. *Archives of Sexual Behavior*, **8**, 379–383.

Routledge, C., Abeyta, A. A. & Roylance, C. (2016) An Existential Function of Evil: The Effects of Religiosity and Compromised Meaning on Belief in Magical Evil Forces. *Motivation and Emotion*, **40**, 681–688.

Rowan, K. & Dwyer, K. (2015) Demonic Possession and Deliverance in the Diaspora: Phenomenological Descriptions from Pentecostal Deliverees. *Mental Health, Religion and Culture*, **18**, 440–455.

Royal Australian and New Zealand College of Psychiatrists (2018) *Position Statement 96: The Relevance of Religion and Spirituality to Psychiatric Practice*. Melbourne, VIC: Royal Australian and New Zealand College of Psychiatrists.

Royal College of Psychiatrists (2013) *Recommendations for Psychiatrists on Spirituality and Religion*. London: Royal College of Psychiatrists.

Royal College of Psychiatrists (2017) *Core Values for Psychiatrists*. London: Royal College of Psychiatrists.

Royal College of Psychiatrists (2022) *Psychiatry Silver Guide: Guidance for Psychiatric Training in the UK, Version 1.0*. London: Royal College of Psychiatrists. silver-guide-final_7–1-22.pdf.

Royal College of Psychiatrists (2024) Exploring Spirituality with People Who Use Mental Health Services. RCPsych eLearning Hub. https://elearninghub.rcpsych.ac.uk/products/Exploring_spirituality_in_mental_health_services.

Rubinstein, J. (1984) Spirit Possession as a Cause of Illness among English Spiritualists. *Cambridge Journal of Anthropology*, **9**, 12–33.

Ruiz-Moral, R. (2022) The 'Medical Friendship' or the True Meaning of the Doctor-Patient Relationship from Two Complementary Perspectives: Goya and Lain. *Medicine, Health Care and Philosophy*, **25**, 111–117.

Ryrie, A. (2012) *The Prayer of Silence*. Oxford: SLG Press.

Sahdan, Z., Pain, R. & McEwan, C. (2021) Demonic Possession: Narratives of Domestic Abuse and Trauma in Malaysia. *Transactions of the Institute of British Geographers*, **47**, 286–301.

Sanchez, A. (2023) Hospital Chaplains: Unfair, Unevidenced, Unnecessary? National Secular Society, 20 April. www.secularism.org.uk/opinion/2023/04/hospital-chaplains-unfair-unevidenced-unnecessary.

Sandage, S. J., Jankowski, P. J., Paine, D. R., Exline, J. J., Ruffing, E. G., Rupert, D., Stavros, G. S. & Bronstein, M. (2020) Testing a Relational Spiritual Model of Psychotherapy Clients' Preferences and Functioning. *Journal of Spirituality in Mental Health*, **24**, 1–21.

Sanderson, A. (2023) *Psychiatry and the Spirit World: True Stories on the Survival of Consciousness after Death*. Rochester, VT: Park Street Press.

Sapkota, R. P., Gurung, D., Neupane, D., Shah, S. K., Kienzler, H. & Kirmayer, L. J. (2014) A Village Possessed by 'Witches': A Mixed-Methods Case-Control Study of Possession and Common Mental Disorders in Rural Nepal. *Culture, Medicine, and Psychiatry*, **38**, 642–668.

Sar, V., Alioglu, F. & Akyuz, G. (2014) Experiences of Possession and Paranormal Phenomena among Women in the General Population: Are They Related to Traumatic Stress and Dissociation? *Journal of Trauma Dissociation*, **15**, 303–318.

Savage, G. H. (2018) Henry Maudsley, MD, FRCPLond., LIDEdin. (Hon.). *Journal of Mental Science*, **64**, 116–129.

Schaap-Jonker, H., Eurelings-Bontekoe, E., Verhagen, P. J. & Zock, H. (2002) Image of God and Personality Pathology: An Exploratory Study among Psychiatric Patients. *Mental Health, Religion and Culture*, **5**, 55–71.

Schjoedt, U., Stodkilde-Jorgensen, H., Geertz, A. W. & Roepstorff, A. (2009) Highly Religious Participants Recruit Areas of Social Cognition in Personal Prayer. *Social Cognitive and Affective Neuroscience*, **4**, 199–207.

Schumann, C., Stroppa, A. & Moreira-Almeida, A. (2011) The Contribution of Faith-Based Health Organisations to Public Health. *International Psychiatry*, **8**, 62–64.

Selberg, T. (2001) Ideas about the Past and Tradition in the Discourse about Neo-Shamanism in a Norwegian Context. *Acta Ethnographica Hungarica*, **46**, 65–74.

Selberg, T. (2010) Journeys, Religion and Authenticity Revisited. In Knudsen, B. T. & Waade, A. M. (Eds.), *Re-investing Authenticity: Tourism, Place and Emotions*. Bristol: Channel View, 228–240.

Shafran, R. & Rachman, S. (2004) Thought-Action Fusion: A Review. *Journal of Behavior Therapy and Experimental Psychiatry*, **35**, 87–107.

Sharp, S. (2012) Prayer Utterances as Aligning Actions. *Journal for the Scientific Study of Religion*, **51**, 257–265.

Shaw, A., Joseph, S. & Linley, P. A. (2005) Religion, Spirituality, and Posttraumatic Growth: A Systematic Review. *Mental Health, Religion and Culture*, **8**, 1–11.

Shidhaye, R. & Vankar, G. K. (2011) Prevalence of Traditional Healing Practices in Psychiatric Outpatients. *Archives of Indian Psychiatry*, **13**, 20–26.

Shooter, M. (1999) Proposal for a Special Interest Group in Spirituality and Psychiatry. *Psychiatric Bulletin*, **23**, 310.

Shuman, J. J. & Meador, K. G. (2003) *Heal Thyself: Spirituality, Medicine, and the Distortion of Christianity*. Oxford: Oxford University Press.

Silton, N. R., Flannelly, K. J., Galek, K. & Ellison, C. G. (2014) Beliefs about God and Mental Health among American Adults. *Journal of Religion and Health*, **53**, 1285–1296.

Simmons, J. A. (2021) Religious, but Not Spiritual: A Constructive Proposal. *Religions*, **12**(6), 433.

Sims, A. (2016) Psychopathology and the Clinical Story. In Cook, C. C. H., Powell, A. & Sims, A. (Eds.), *Spirituality and Narrative in Psychiatric Practice*. London: Royal College of Psychiatrists, 25–38.

Sims, A. C. P. (1988) The Psychiatrist as Priest. *Journal of the Royal Society for the Promotion of Health*, **108**, 160–163.

Singh, S. P. (2023) Sakshi and Dhyana: The Origin of Mindfulness-Based Therapies. *BJPsych Bulletin*, **47**, 94–97.

Slominski, K. L., Powell, A. J. & Cook, C. C. H. (Eds.) (2026) *The Routledge Handbook of Spirituality, Religion, and Medical Humanities.* London: Routledge.

Smith, K. (2012) From Dividual and Individual Selves to Porous Subjects. *Australasian Journal of Anthropology*, 23, 50–64.

Somer, E. (2004) Trance Possession Disorder in Judaism: Sixteenth-Century Dybbuks in the Near East. *Journal of Trauma and Dissociation*, 5, 131–146.

Speeth, K. R. (1982) On Psychotherapeutic Attention. *Journal of Transpersonal Psychology*, 14, 141–160.

Spencer, W. (2010) To Absent Friends: Classical Spiritualist Mediumship and New Age Channelling Compared and Contrasted. *Journal of Contemporary Religion*, 16, 343–360.

Spiro, M. E. (1993) Is the Western Conception of the Self 'Peculiar' within the Context of the World Cultures? *Ethos*, 21, 107–153.

Stauner, N., Exline, J. J. & Wilt, J. A. (2020) Meaning, Religious/Spiritual Struggles, and Well-Being. In Vail III, K. E. & Routledge, C. (Eds.), *The Science of Religion, Spirituality, and Existentialism*. London: Academic Press, 287–303.

Steger, M. F. (2022) Meaning in Life is a Fundamental Protective Factor in the Context of Psychopathology. *World Psychiatry*, 21, 389–390.

Stephenson, C. E. (2017) *Possession: Jung's Comparative Anatomy of the Psyche.* London: Routledge.

Stevens, A. (1999) *On Jung.* Harmondsworth: Penguin.

Stevens, A. (2001) *Jung: A Very Short Introduction.* Oxford: Oxford University Press.

Stöckigt, B., Jeserich, F., Walach, H., Elies, M., Brinkhaus, B. & Teut, M. (2021) Experiences and Perceived Effects of Rosary Praying: A Qualitative Study. *Journal of Religion and Health*, 60, 3886–3906.

Stone, C. B., Coman, A., Brown, A. D., Koppel, J. & Hirst, W. (2012) Toward a Science of Silence: The Consequences of Leaving a Memory Unsaid. *Perspectives on Psychological Science*, 7, 39–53.

Storr, A. (2001) *Freud: A Very Short Introduction.* Oxford: Oxford University Press.

Stoyanov, D., Machamer, P. & Schaffner, K. F. (2013) In Quest for Scientific Psychiatry: Toward Bridging the Explanatory Gap. *Philosophy, Psychiatry, and Psychology*, 20, 261–273.

Suhail, K. & Cochrane, R. (2002) Effect of Culture and Environment on the Phenomenology of Delusions and Hallucinations. *International Journal of Social Psychiatry*, 48, 126–138.

Szasz, T. (2008) *Psychiatry: The Science of Lies.* Syracuse, NY: Syracuse University Press.

Szasz, T. S. (1962) *The Myth of Mental Illness.* London: Granada.

Ta, T. M. T., Boge, K., Cao, T. D., Schomerus, G., Nguyen, T. D., Dettling, M., Mungee, A., Martensen, L. K., Diefenbacher, A., Angermeyer, M. C. & Hahn, E. (2018) Public Attitudes towards Psychiatrists in the Metropolitan Area of Hanoi, Vietnam. *Asian Journal of Psychiatry*, 32, 44–49.

Tait, R., Currier, J. M. & Harris, J. I. (2016) Prayer Coping, Disclosure of Trauma, and Mental Health Symptoms among Recently Deployed United States Veterans of the Iraq and Afghanistan Conflicts. *International Journal for the Psychology of Religion*, 26, 31–45.

Tajima-Pozo, K., Zambrano-Enriquez, D., De Anta, L., Moron, M. D., Carrasco, J. L., Lopez-Ibor, J. J. & Diaz-Marsa, M. (2011) Practicing Exorcism in Schizophrenia. *British Medical Journal Case Reports*, 2011, bcr1020092350.

Tatala, M. & Wojtasiński, M. (2021) The Validity of Prayer Importance Scale (PIS). *Religions*, 12(11), 1032.

Taves, A. (2011) Special Things as Building Blocks of Religions. In Orsi, R. A. (Ed.), *The Cambridge Companion to Religious Studies*. Cambridge: Cambridge University Press, 58–83.

Taylor, C. (2007) *A Secular Age.* Cambridge, MA: Belknap Press.

Teja, J. S., Khanna, B. S. & Subrahmanyam, T. B. (1970) 'Possession States' in Indian Patients. *Indian Journal of Psychiatry*, **12**, 71–87.

Tepper, L., Rogers, S. A., Coleman, E. M. & Malony, H. N. (2001) The Prevalence of Religious Coping among Persons with Persistent Mental Illness. *Psychiatric Services*, **52**, 660–665.

Thalbourne, M. A. & Delin, P. S. (1994) A Common Thread Underlying Belief in the Paranormal, Creative Personality, Mystical Experience and Psychopathology. *Journal of Parapsychology*, **58**, 3–38.

Thalbourne, M. A. & Maltby, J. (2008) Transliminality, Thin Boundaries, Unusual Experiences, and Temporal Lobe Lability. *Personality and Individual Differences*, **44**, 1617–1623.

Thomas, P. & Bracken, P. (2018) Critical Psychiatry in Practice. *Advances in Psychiatric Treatment*, **10**, 361–370.

Thomason, T. C. (2010) Psychological Treatments to Avoid. *Alabama Counseling Association Journal*, **36**, 39–48.

Trammel, R. C. (2017) A Phenomenological Study of Christian Practitioners Who Use Mindfulness. *Journal of Spirituality in Mental Health*, **20**, 199–224.

Tripathi, V., Devaney, K. J., Lazar, S. W. & Somers, D. C. (2024) Silence Practice Modulates the Resting State Functional Connectivity of Language Network with Default Mode and Dorsal Attention Networks in Long-Term Meditators. *Mindfulness*, **15**, 665–674.

Tung, E. S., Ruffing, E. G., Paine, D. R., Jankowski, P. J. & Sandage, S. J. (2017) Attachment to God as Mediator of the Relationship between God Representations and Mental Health. *Journal of Spirituality in Mental Health*, **20**, 95–113.

Turner, T. (1988) Henry Maudsley – Psychiatrist, Philosopher and Entrepreneur. *Psychological Medicine*, **18**, 551–574.

Tyler, P. (2014) Mindfulness, Heartfulness, or Soulfulness? Teresa of Avila, Otto Rank, James Hillman and the Return of the Soul. *Milltown Studies*, **74**, 27–50.

Tyler, P. (2018) *Christian Mindfulness: Theology and Practice*. London: SCM.

UK Council for Psychotherapy (2014) *Conversion Therapy: Consensus Statement*. London: UK Council for Psychotherapy.

Ulanov, A. & Ulanov, B. (1985) *Primary Speech: A Psychology of Prayer*. London: SCM.

Upenieks, L. (2023) Unpacking the Relationship between Prayer and Anxiety: A Consideration of Prayer Types and Expectations in the United States. *Journal of Religion and Health*, **62**, 1810–1831.

Utsch, M., Anderssen-Reuster, U., Frick, E., Gross, W., Murken, S., Schouler-Ocak, M. & Stotz-Ingenlath, G. (2017) Empfehlungen zum Umgang mit Religiosität und Spiritualität in Psychiatrie und Psychotherapie. *Spiritual Care*, **6**, 141–146.

Vaillant, G. E. (2013) Psychiatry, Religion, Positive Emotions and Spirituality. *Asian Journal of Psychiatry*, **6**, 590–594.

Van Der Hart, O., Lierens, R. & Goodwin, J. (1996) Jeanne Fery: A Sixteenth-Century Case of Dissociative Identity Disorder. *Journal of Psychohistory*, **24**, 18–35.

Van Nieuw Amerongen-Meeuse, J. C., Schaap-Jonker, H., Schuhmann, C., Anbeek, C. & Braam, A. W. (2019) The 'Religiosity Gap' in a Clinical Setting: Experiences of Mental Health Care Consumers and Professionals. *Mental Health, Religion and Culture*, **21**, 737–752.

Van Nieuw Amerongen-Meeuse, J. C., Braam, A. W., Anbeek, C. & Schaap-Jonker, H. (2020) 'Beyond Boundaries or Best Practice' Prayer in Clinical Mental Health Care: Opinions of Professionals and Patients. *Religions*, **11**(10), 492.

Van Tongeren, D. R., Sanders, M., Edwards, M., Davis, E. B., Aten, J. D., Ranter, J. M., Tsarouhis, A., Short, A., Cuthbert, A., Hook, J. N. & Davis, D. E. (2019) Religious and Spiritual Struggles Alter God Representations. *Psychology of Religion and Spirituality*, **11**, 225–232.

Van Uden, M. H. F. & Zondag, H. J. (2011) Still Knockin' on Heaven's Door: Narcissism and Prayer. *Journal of Empirical Theology*, **24**, 19–35.

Varma, L. P., Srivastava, D. K. & Sahay, R. N. (1970) Possession Syndrome. *Indian Journal of Psychiatry*, **12**, 58–70.

Vinogradov, A. (2008) 'After the Past, before the Present': New Shamanism in Gorny Altai. *Anthropology of Consciousness*, **10**, 36–44.

Vitorino, L. M., Lucchetti, G., Leao, F. C., Vallada, H., Peres, M. F. P. (2018) The Association between Spirituality and Religiousness and Mental Health. *Scientific Reports*, **8**(1), 17233.

Walker, G. C. (2000) Secular Eschatology: Beliefs about Afterlife. *OMEGA*, **41**, 5–22.

Walliss, J. (2001) Continuing Bonds: Relationships between the Living and the Dead within Contemporary Spiritualism. *Mortality*, **6**, 127–145.

Weatherhead, S. & Daiches, A. (2010) Muslim Views on Mental Health and Psychotherapy. *Psychology and Psychotherapy*, **83**, 75–89.

Weber, S. R., Pargament, K. I., Kunik, M. E., Lomax II, J. W. & Stanley, M. A. (2012) Psychological Distress among Religious Nonbelievers: A Systematic Review. *Journal of Religion and Health*, **51**, 72–86.

Webster, R. (2005) *Why Freud Was Wrong: Sin, Science and Psychoanalysis*. Oxford: Orwell Press.

Weil, S. (1952) *Gravity and Grace*. London: Routledge & Kegan Paul.

Weisberg, B. (2005) *Talking to the Dead: Kate and Maggie Fox and the Rise of Spiritualism*. New York: HarperCollins.

Whitwell, F. D. & Barker, M. G. (1980) 'Possession' in Psychiatric Patients in Britain. *British Journal of Medical Psychology*, **53**, 287–295.

Wield, C. (2012) *A Thorn in My Mind: Mental Illness, Stigma and the Church*. Watford: Instant Apostle.

Williams, R. (2012) *Faith in the Public Square*. London: Bloomsbury.

Winkeljohn Black, S., Pössel, P., Jeppsen, B. D., Bjerg, A. C. & Wooldridge, D. T. (2015) Disclosure during Private Prayer as a Mediator between Prayer Type and Mental Health in an Adult Christian Sample. *Journal of Religion and Health*, **54**, 540–553.

Winkeljohn Black, S., Pössel, P., Rosmarin, D. H., Tariq, A. & Jeppsen, B. D. (2017) Prayer Type, Disclosure, and Mental Health across Religious Groups. *Counseling and Values*, **62**, 216–234.

Winnicott, D. W. (1982) *The Maturational Processes and the Facilitating Environment*. London: Hogarth Press.

Wirzba, N. (2006) Attention and Responsibility: The Work of Prayer. In Benson, B. E. & Wirzba, N. (Eds.), *The Phenomenology of Prayer*. New York: Fordham University Press, 88–100.

Wong-McDonald, A. & Gorsuch, R. L. (2000) Surrender to God: An Additional Coping Style? *Journal of Psychology and Theology*, **28**, 149–161.

Woods, A., Jones, N., Alderson-Day, B., Callard, F. & Fernyhough, C. (2015) Experiences of Hearing Voices: Analysis of a Novel Phenomenological Survey. *The Lancet Psychiatry*, **2**(4), 323–331.

Woods, A., Alderson-Day, B. & Fernyhough, C. (2022) Voices in Psychosis: Interdisciplinary Listening. In Woods, A., Alderson-Day, B. & Fernyhough, C. (Eds.), *Voices in Psychosis: Interdisciplinary Perspectives*. Oxford: Oxford University Press, 3–16.

Worthington, E. L. Jr, Hook, J. N., Davis, D. E. & McDaniel, M. A. (2011) Religion and Spirituality. *Journal of Clinical Psychology*, **67**, 204–214.

Wright, P. (2014) Lay Christian Understanding of Sin: A Qualitative Study and Appraisal of the 'Ordinary Theology' of an Anglican Congregation. *Theology and Ministry*, **3**, 1–11.

Wynaden, D., Chapman, R., Orb, A., McGowan, S., Zeeman, Z. & Yeak, S. (2005) Factors That Influence Asian Communities' Access to Mental Health Care. *International Journal of Mental Health Nursing*, **14**, 88–95.

Yangarber-Hicks, N. (2004) Religious Coping Styles and Recovery from Serious Mental Illness. *Journal of Psychology and Theology*, **32**, 305–317.

Yap, P. M. (1960) The Possession Syndrome: A Comparison of Hong Kong and French

Findings. *Journal of Mental Science*, **106**, 114–137.

Yoon, J. D., Shin, J. H., Nian, A. L. & Curlin, F. A. (2015) Religion, Sense of Calling, and the Practice of Medicine: Findings from a National Survey of Primary Care Physicians and Psychiatrists. *Southern Medical Journal*, **108**(3), 189–195.

Zaleski, P. & Zaleski, C. (2005) *Prayer: A History.* Boston, MA: Houghton Mifflin.

Zeiger, R. B. (2022) Honi the Circle-Maker: An Ancient Narrative for Creating Temenos in Challenging Times. *Innovation: The European Journal of Social Science Research*, **36**, 141–154.

Zhang, D., Lee, E. K. P., Mak, E. C. W., Ho, C. Y. & Wong, S. Y. S. (2021) Mindfulness-Based Interventions: An Overall Review. *British Medical Bulletin*, **138**, 41–57.

Zieger, A., Mungee, A., Schomerus, G., Ta, T. M. T., Weyers, A., Boge, K., Dettling, M., Bajbouj, M., Von Lersner, U., Angermeyer, M. C., Tandon, A. & Hahn, E. (2017) Attitude toward Psychiatrists and Psychiatric Medication: A Survey from Five Metropolitan Cities in India. *Indian Journal of Psychiatry*, **59**, 341–346.

Zondag, H. J. & Uden, M. H. F. V. (2014) 'My Special Prayer': On Self, God and Prayer. *European Journal of Mental Health*, **9**, 3–19.

Index

For EU product safety concerns, contact us at Calle de José Abascal, 56–1°, 28003 Madrid, Spain or eugpsr@cambridge.org.

www.ingramcontent.com/pod-product-compliance
Ingram Content Group UK Ltd.
Pitfield, Milton Keynes, MK11 3LW, UK
UKHW022050020626
471784UK00008B/322